Diagnostic Imaging for Pharmacists

Notices

Diagnostic Imaging for Pharmacists

Edited by

Blaine Templar Smith, BSPharm, PhD
Past Chair, Department of Pharmaceutical Sciences
Saint Joseph College School of Pharmacy
Hartford, Connecticut

Kara D. Weatherman, PharmD, BCNP, FAPhA
Clinical Assistant Professor of Pharmacy Practice
Purdue University
West Lafayette, Indiana

American Pharmacists Association®
Improving medication use. Advancing patient care.
APhA
Washington, D.C.

Editor: Nancy Tarleton Landis
Acquiring Editor: Sandra J. Cannon
Cover Design: Scott Neitzke, APhA Creative Services
Composition: Circle Graphics
Proofreading: Kathleen K. Wolter
Indexing: Jen Burton, Columbia Indexing Group

Published by the American Pharmacists Association
2215 Constitution Avenue, N.W., Washington, DC 20037-2985
www.pharmacist.com www.pharmacylibrary.com

APhA was founded in 1852 as the American Pharmaceutical Association.

To comment on this book via e-mail, send your message to the publisher at aphabooks@aphanet.org.

Library of Congress Cataloging-in-Publication Data

Diagnostic imaging for pharmacists / edited by Blaine Templar Smith, Kara D. Weatherman.
p. ; cm.
Includes bibliographical references and index.
ISBN 978-1-58212-153-6
I. Smith, Blaine T. II. Weatherman, Kara D. (Kara Duncan) III. American Pharmacists Association.
[DNLM: 1. Radiopharmaceuticals—diagnostic use. 2. Contrast Media—diagnostic use. 3. Diagnostic Imaging—methods. 4. Nuclear Medicine. 5. Pharmacy. WN 445]

616.07′575—dc23

2011041755

How to Order This Book
Online: www.pharmacist.com/shop_apha
By phone: 800-878-0729 (770-280-0085 from outside the United States)
VISA®, MasterCard®, and American Express® cards accepted

Contents

Preface

Diagnostic imaging is an essential part of medical care today. Pharmacists, who are integral members of the health care team, historically have had very little involvement in this area of practice, other than to recognize that imaging procedures may directly dictate a patient's pharmacologic treatment plan. Few practicing pharmacists have a high level of comfort with issues related to diagnostic imaging, because most schools of pharmacy do not cover this area to any appreciable extent in their curricula. Patients undergoing diagnostic imaging often receive a variety of pharmaceutical agents as part of the imaging procedure, and these agents have historically been overseen by the radiology department instead of the pharmacy department. However, with recent changes in regulatory oversight of medication management and with increased attention to this area by accreditation bodies, pharmacists are finding that they need a better understanding of policies and procedures for the use of pharmacologic agents in diagnostic imaging. Most practitioners are forced to gain this knowledge on the job or by conducting their own searches for available information, very little of which has been directly aimed toward the pharmacy community.

It is for these reasons that this book came to fruition. The book's primary focus is on the pharmaceutical agents used in the imaging suite—contrast agents in x-ray, magnetic resonance imaging (MRI), and ultrasound; radiopharmaceuticals in nuclear medicine and positron emission tomography; and traditional pharmaceuticals that are used as interventional agents during various imaging procedures. To supplement pharmacists' knowledge about the imaging modalities themselves, enabling them to better understand and participate in patient care, we have included basic chapters on each type of imaging modality (x-ray, MRI, ultrasound, and nuclear medicine). Finally, we have included a discussion of the regulatory oversight of diagnostic imaging and the safety procedures that govern the use of ionizing radiation.

It is our hope that this book will provide practitioners with a basic understanding of diagnostic imaging and the pharmaceuticals used as part of the imaging process. The pharmacy community should embrace this opportunity to move into a new area of practice. Pharmacists' increased level of expertise in pharmaceutical use in diagnostic imaging can only serve to improve overall patient care.

Acknowledgments

We wish to express our great appreciation to the many contributors, proofreaders, and American Pharmacists Association staff members who helped bring this book to fruition. It was not without many challenges—and thus triumphs—that the task was completed. As editors, we thank the authors for their patience through each change and iteration that was requested and for their willingness to make the changes without the benefit of seeing the "big picture" we were trying to achieve.

We thank each of the authors for taking the time and effort to provide us with an exceptional body of work. Thank you for withstanding the sometimes-withering requests made of you. You can be proud of the product we have created!

To Joan Templar Smith, PhD, for impeccable and timely editing work and to Ross Weatherman, PhD, who acted as a sounding board, provided impromptu editing and consulting, and provided support during the entire process, we both express our gratitude for your involvement in this project. We are also thankful to Sandy Cannon and the staff at APhA for being confident, patient, and helpful all along the way, even as we began to run late.

We, the editors, were contributors, guides, and conduits, but all the contributors together made the product what it is, requiring very minor interference from either of us, which made our job much easier! Once again, our thanks to you all and congratulations on a job well done!

Blaine Templar Smith
Kara Duncan Weatherman

November 2011

Contributors

Sam Baird, MD
Associate Professor of Radiology
Department of Radiologic Sciences
University of Oklahoma Health Sciences Center
Oklahoma City, Oklahoma

Allegra L. DePietro, BSPharm, MS, BCNP
Nuclear Pharmacy Manager
Division of Nuclear Medicine and Molecular Imaging
Massachusetts General Hospital
Boston, Massachusetts

Cory Duncan, MD
Emergency Medicine Physician
Arlington Memorial Hospital
Arlington, Texas

Wendy Galbraith, PharmD, BCNP
Clinical Assistant Professor
University of Oklahoma Health Sciences Center Nuclear Pharmacy
University of Oklahoma College of Pharmacy
Oklahoma City, Oklahoma

Vivian S. Loveless, PharmD, BCNP, FAPhA
Associate Professor, Department of Pharmaceutical Sciences
University of Tennessee Health Science Center
Memphis, Tennessee

Hal J. Minnigan, MD, PhD, RDMS
Assistant Professor of Clinical Emergency Medicine
Coordinator of Ultrasound Education
Department of Emergency Medicine
Indiana University School of Medicine
Indianapolis, Indiana

Mack L. Richard, MS, CHP
Radiation Safety Officer
Indiana University School of Medicine
Indianapolis, Indiana

Brian Schumer, PharmD
Western Area Vice President
Triad Isotopes, Inc.
Houston, Texas

Blaine Templar Smith, BSPharm, PhD
Past Chair, Department of Pharmaceutical Sciences
Saint Joseph College School of Pharmacy
Hartford, Connecticut

Jessica Turner, PharmD
Cardinal Health Fellow—Clinical Nuclear Pharmacy and Radiopharmaceutical Safety
Purdue University
West Lafayette, Indiana

Kara D. Weatherman, PharmD, BCNP, FAPhA
Clinical Assistant Professor of Pharmacy Practice
Purdue University
West Lafayette, Indiana

Dee H. Wu, PhD
Chief, Technology Applications and Translational Research
Associate Professor
Department of Radiological Sciences
University of Oklahoma Health Sciences Center
Oklahoma City, Oklahoma

CHAPTER 1

Diagnostic Imaging and the Role of the Pharmacist

Kara D. Weatherman

Radiology is the area of medical practice that focuses on visualization of the interior of the human body through the use of various imaging technologies. Although this medical specialty has essentially been in existence since Wilhelm Roentgen published his work on x-rays in 1895, it is an area of practice that most pharmacists are rarely if ever exposed to during their academic training. In recent years, however, there has been increasing interest in pharmacist involvement in the radiology department, not from the perspective of the imaging modalities themselves but because of the widespread use of pharmaceuticals as adjunct agents in the acquisition of diagnostic imaging data. As the number of patients who undergo diagnostic imaging procedures increases, so does the number who are exposed to pharmaceuticals used to augment the data obtained through imaging. In some cases, as in nuclear medicine, the imaging procedure is entirely dependent on the administration of pharmaceutical agents. In other cases, as in x-ray and magnetic resonance imaging, pharmaceuticals are administered to provide various levels of contrast between the organs and vessels of the body, allowing a clearer picture of the complex anatomy being studied. Many of the pharmaceutical agents being used carry specific risks to patients; these risks must be understood, anticipated, and addressed when the drugs are administered. In addition, like any pharmaceutical product administered to patients, these agents have the potential to create adverse reactions that should be monitored and reported.

Pharmacists' unique knowledge and understanding of drug therapy makes them the most logical providers of drug information related to diagnostic imaging. Historically, however, the role of the pharmacist in the radiology department has ranged from limited to nonexistent. As we will discuss, the control of all pharmaceuticals administered in this environment has usually fallen within the scope of medical practice of the radiologist, who ordered and administered the agents, and the use of these agents has been considered part of the imaging test rather than separate medication administration. With today's emphasis on medication therapy management (MTM) and pharmacists' expanding responsibility for providing this type of drug review, the administration of pharmaceutical agents in the radiology department should not be excluded. In some institutions pharmacists are becoming involved in the radiology department, but many pharmacists still are uncomfortable working with a class of drugs about which they generally know so little. It is our hope that this publication will assist practitioners who find their professional responsibilities expanding to include the area of radiology and radiologic pharmaceuticals.

Radiology

The four main areas of diagnostic radiology are x-ray, magnetic resonance imaging (MRI), ultrasound, and nuclear medicine. Within each of these areas are many different types of studies. For example, fluoroscopy is a type of x-ray study in which multiple x-rays are taken in rapid sequence to show movement within the body. In nuclear medicine, both single-photon emission computed tomography (SPECT) and positron emission tomography (PET) use radioactive pharmaceuticals to provide diagnostic information about various physiologic processes within the body. Each of the subspecialties is discussed in detail in the chapter on that specific imaging modality. The American College of Radiology recently estimated that more than 570 million medical imaging procedures are performed in the United States each year.[1] Adjunct pharmaceuticals play a role in many of these studies, either as essential components of the imaging study or to enhance the information obtained. In x-ray, ultrasound, and MRI imaging, the pharmaceuticals used are called contrast agents because they enhance the contrast between various tissues, allowing better visualization of abnormalities within a field of tissues that radiographically look very similar. In nuclear medicine, the radioactive molecule being imaged is introduced into the body in the form of a radiopharmaceutical, while other nonradioactive agents are used to enhance the information obtained.

In most institutions, all aspects of the use of pharmaceuticals in radiology departments fall under the oversight of the radiology department staff rather than the pharmacy staff. Many institutional pharmacy departments have considered the administration of radiologic pharmaceuticals to fall within the radiologist's scope of practice, since most radiology-specific agents have no use outside the imaging suite. Often, oversight of the use of these agents has been passed on to the radiologic technologists who actually perform the imaging procedures, usually under a protocol reviewed and approved by the staff radiologists. Traditional pharmaceuticals that are used to enhance some imaging studies have provided the only link between many radiology departments and the in-house pharmacy department, with the pharmacy supplying these drugs to radiology in small quantities or on an as-needed basis to ensure maximum utilization of the products. This traditional arrangement has assumed that all pre-administration medication reviews and adverse drug reaction monitoring and reporting will be coordinated by the radiology staff.

The administration of pharmaceuticals in the radiology department is not without problems. As you will see in the individual chapters on the pharmaceuticals used for each imaging modality, some of these agents have the potential to cause severe and even fatal adverse reactions. In addition, these agents may be misused, as a result of variations in training, varying levels of staff experience, fatigue, increasing diversity of the patient population, increasing complexity of medical procedures and technologies, poor communication, poor reporting systems, reliance on automated systems, and increasing time constraints. In 2006, the United States Pharmacopeia Center for the Advancement of Patient Safety issued a report titled "Medication Errors in Radiological Service Areas."[2] Data for the report were collected over a 5-year period from 315 different radiology sites. A total of 2032 errors were identified, 56.8% of which occurred in the diagnostic radiology suite. Of these errors, 81.1% actually reached the patient, and 12% caused some level of patient harm. The report identified several factors that contributed to these errors: limited published data on medication errors in this practice site, a lack of communication and lack of patient information being passed on to the radiology staff, and a system focused more on the imaging procedure than on the patient.

Medication Therapy Management

MTM was introduced as a result of the Medicare Prescription Drug Improvement and Modernization Act of 2003 (MMA).[3] This act of Congress created several benefits that had direct applicability to pharmacy, including the Medicare Part D drug benefit and health savings accounts, and it defined the tenets of MTM. A major focus of the MMA was to ensure that Medicare patients being treated for chronic diseases with pharmaceuticals covered under Part D were using these medications appropriately to improve therapeutic outcomes and decrease the risk of adverse events. Since MMA did not explicitly define what services would be provided as part of medication review, 11 key pharmacy organizations collaborated to create and support a definition of MTM and outline the services considered to be within the scope of this type of review. This definition was approved July 27, 2004.[4]

MTM has five core elements: medication therapy review, a personal medication record, a medication-related action plan, intervention and/or referral, and documentation and follow-up.[4] Each of these elements is discussed below.

Medication Therapy Review (MTR)

MTR is a systematic process for collecting patient information, assessing the patient's current medication therapies to determine if any medication-related problems exist, developing a prioritized list of medication-related problems, and then creating a plan to resolve the problems. The pharmacist initially performs a comprehensive review of the patient's drug therapy and then works with the patient, the primary care physician, and other health care professionals to resolve any issues that arise. In addition, targeted reviews can be performed to identify how any new drug added to the patient's regimen fits into the comprehensive MTR. If drug-specific problems arise, targeted reviews can be used to address these issues in the context of the patient's complete medication history.

Personal Medication Record (PMR)

One benefit of performing the MTR is that a PMR can be generated. The PMR is a complete record of the patient's medications, including both prescription and nonprescription or over-the-counter products, herbals, and dietary supplements. A PMR should be a dynamic, ideally electronic document that is updated each time a medication change occurs. A PMR should be written at a level that a patient would understand and should include patient-specific information (e.g., name and date of birth), contact information for each prescribing physician and the pharmacist who created the PMR, patient allergies, and medication-related issues. For each medication the patient is taking, the drug, indication, instructions for use, start date, projected stop date (if known), and any special instructions should be listed. Patients should be able to carry the PMR with them at all times and provide it to any new medical professional as a complete summary of all their pharmaceutical needs.

Medication-Related Action Plan (MAP)

The MAP is a patient-focused document that details how patients should be tracking their progress as part of a self-management program. A major goal of MTM is for patients to become an active part of the process and take partial responsibility for the success of their drug therapy. The MAP lists items for the patient to work on between health care visits.

Intervention and Referral

In this element of MTM, the pharmacist provides consultation and attempts to address any medication-related problems that were identified in the MTR. The pharmacist may need to intervene on the patient's behalf by communicating with physicians or other health care professionals and suggesting methods to address the identified problems.

Documentation and Follow-up

The pharmacist should document all services and interventions provided in the process of monitoring and evaluating patients' medication therapy. In addition, over time, thorough documentation will provide the pharmacist with a mechanism for billing for the services provided.

MTM in Radiology

A major concern with MTM in the radiology department is how to merge it with the standard dispensing and administration practices used in radiology departments for many years. This is not an insignificant problem, and it has created some issues in radiology departments as pharmacy departments have become more interested in the pharmaceuticals used in imaging procedures. Unfortunately, radiology does not fit easily into the standard MTM mold.

One issue is how radiology products fit into the MTR process. MTM is intended to be performed mainly to evaluate drug therapy for chronic diseases. For most patients, pharmaceuticals administered in a radiology department are single administrations that may or may not be repeated at some point, depending on whether the patients require additional radiology exams during their lifetime. Radiology administration records may not be readily available to the pharmacist performing MTR, and it is unlikely that a patient who reports problems with radiology-based pharmaceuticals would have enough information about the agents used to provide an adequate description of the medication-related problem.

The PMR is probably the most useful part of MTM in a radiology department, since it provides an up-to-date document that can be reviewed prior to administration of any pharmaceutical to identify potential interactions or adverse reactions to the radiologic pharmaceutical. This works well only if the person who reviews the PMR is able to interpret the information and make correlations with the drug product that the patient will be receiving in the radiology department. Many radiology technologists do not have strong training in pharmaceuticals used outside radiology departments. Although they may be familiar with radiologic pharmaceuticals, they may not be comfortable reviewing a patient's PMR and making judgments about whether the patient is a candidate for receiving the radiologic pharmaceutical. Under the scope of MTM, any *licensed* health care professional can perform this function, so it would fall to the physician in the department to provide the MTM review.

Unfortunately, the PMR does not lend itself to including single-administration pharmaceuticals. It is designed to be a summary of the patient's current drug therapy. Any single-administration dose would be on the PMR only at the time of administration and then would immediately be removed. Including every single-administration agent on the PMR would quickly make it a very cumbersome document, limiting its usefulness. However, not having these single-administration agents on the PMR contributes to the difficulty of keeping track of adverse reactions to these agents. Although adverse reactions and major issues with a radiologic pharmaceutical could be noted on the PMR, making an addition to the patient's PMR would require accessing the original data and possibly reporting outside the institution, which would require time and effort on the part of the radiology staff. It is easy to see how minor problems could go unreported, but a minor problem can be a precursor to more severe problems with subsequent administrations.

Most radiology departments have a medication-related action plan in which the technologist gives the patient a spoken explanation of what to look for after the study or a written list of problems that would warrant a phone call to the department should they arise. Patients may not truly understand these instructions; often, patients are feeling stressed about undergoing the imaging procedure, and their instructions may go unheeded. Furthermore, given a complete list of potential side effects and adverse reactions, patients could, through the power of suggestion, believe they are experiencing these effects. Also, since many of the adverse reactions to the pharmaceuticals used in radiology are nonspecific, it would be easy to falsely identify an adverse reaction.

The Joint Commission

For most pharmacists in institutional practice, the primary impetus behind increased pharmacy department involvement in radiology is Joint Commission accreditation status. The Joint Commission requires for accreditation many areas of compliance that affect every hospital department, including radiology. In this book, we will discuss, in relation to the radiology department, Joint Commission requirements related to medication management (MM) and medication-related National Patient Safety Goals. The complexities of the MM standards are beyond the scope of this chapter, but it is important to recognize that the Joint Commission considers all contrast agents and radiopharmaceuticals as medications. The Joint Commission defines a medication as "any product designated by the FDA as a drug, as well as any sample medication, herbal remedies, vitamins, nutraceuticals, over the counter drugs, vaccines, diagnostic and contrast agents, respiratory therapy treatments, parenteral nutrition, blood derivatives and intravenous solutions (plain, with electrolytes and/or drugs)."[5] This ensures that contrast agents and radiopharmaceuticals will have the same level of controls as other medications in the areas of prescribing, dispensing, storage, security, administration, and monitoring of adverse events.

The Joint Commission's MM standard 5.01.01 element of performance (EP) 1 requires that all medication orders or prescriptions be reviewed for appropriateness prior to dispensing. This review is to be performed by a licensed pharmacist unless a licensed independent practitioner (LIP) controls the ordering, preparation, and administration of the medication or unless the medication is urgently needed.[5] Most radiology departments have practiced with the radiologist acting as the LIP. However, in most departments, the radiologist has passed all aspects of administration of contrast agents to the technologist staff, who work under the oversight, but not necessarily under the direct supervision, of the radiology physician. The Joint Commission believes that oversight includes the radiologist remaining with the patient during the administration process unless there has been prior review of the order by a licensed pharmacist. The American College of Radiology objected to this requirement, citing the interruption of workflow and the lack of physician and pharmacist resources to adequately carry out this requirement. In January 2007, the Joint Commission revised this standard, allowing a hospital radiology department to define the role of the LIP in the direct supervision of patients receiving contrast agents and radiopharmaceuticals. This can be done through the development of protocols or policies that clearly state the role of the LIP in direct supervision. The protocol or policy must be approved by the medical staff and must include a definition of the LIP's role in the administration process, ensuring that the LIP will be able to intervene in a timely manner in any case in which the patient experiences any type of adverse reaction due to the administration of the medications used.[6]

The American College of Radiology has issued a document titled "Practice Guidelines for the Use of Intravascular Contrast Media," which the Joint Commission recommends as a reference source for the development of protocols or policies in the area of radiology.[7] The hospital pharmacy staff should also have input in the development of these policies and protocols. However, many pharmacists are uncomfortable providing information regarding these drug products.

Most pharmacy school curricula do not include courses emphasizing contrast agents or radiopharmaceuticals. Since pharmacy staff members lack training in this area, on-the-job training in the practice site is also limited. It generally falls to pharmacists themselves to gain more knowledge of contrast agents and radiopharmaceuticals in order to contribute to medication safety with these agents. It is our hope that this reference will help broaden and deepen the knowledge base of the practicing pharmacists who will be called on to provide this service in their institutions.

Conclusion

As you will see in the following chapters, we have approached this topic with the assumption that many pharmacists have not had this type of training as part of their pharmacy curriculum, nor have they had extensive education on the various diagnostic imaging modalities themselves. We have attempted to provide chapters that discuss in detail the various pharmaceuticals used in each of the different imaging modalities that we believed would be of greatest interest to practicing pharmacists. Furthermore, we believed that a basic understanding of the imaging modalities themselves would help pharmacists better understand the context in which the pharmaceuticals are being used. Thus, we have included an introduction to each imaging modality, followed by a chapter that discusses the specific pharmaceuticals used in that modality. We have also included some background information on ionizing radiation, used in both x-ray and nuclear medicine imaging, to provide additional detail on the risks and concerns associated with the use of radiation in imaging studies. Although this book can be no substitute for the judicious study of the package inserts of the various products, we believe it will provide pharmacists with the basic understanding they require to become more involved in and knowledgeable about this area of practice and the pharmaceuticals used therein.

References

1. American College of Radiology. ACR statement regarding the recent USP study on medication error rates in imaging facilities. January 18, 2006. www.acr.org/MainMenuCategories/media_room/FeaturedCategories/PressReleases/Archive/1182006ACRStatementRegardingtheRecentUSPStudyonMedicationErrorRatesinImagingFacilitiesDoc3.aspx. Accessed August 2010.

2. United States Pharmacopeia. MedMarx data report. A chartbook of 2000–2004 findings from intensive care units and radiological services. 2005:66–112.
3. Medicare Prescription Drug Improvement and Modernization Act of 2003. http://frwebgate.access.gpo.gov/cgi-bin/getdoc.cgi?dbname=108_cong_bills&docid=f:h1enr.txt.pdf. Accessed August 2010.
4. Medication Therapy Management Services Definition and Program Criteria. Approved July 27, 2004. www.accp.com/docs/positions/misc/MTMDefn.pdf.
5. The Joint Commission. *2008 Comprehensive Accreditation Manual for Hospitals: The Official Handbook.* Oakbrook Terrace, IL: Joint Commission Resources; 2008.
6. The Joint Commission. Approved: interim action for standard MM.4.10, element of performance 1, for critical access hospitals and hospitals: modifications for the emergency department and radiology practitioners. *Jt Comm Perspect.* 2007;27:9.
7. American College of Radiology. ACR practice guideline for the use of intravascular contrast media. 2007. www.acr.org/SecondaryMainMenuCategories/quality_safety/guidelines/dx/iv_contrast.aspx. Accessed September 2010.

CHAPTER 2

Introduction to Ionizing Radiation

Blaine Templar Smith

Pharmacists do not usually have training or experience in the methods, techniques, and pharmaceuticals used in diagnostic imaging. Today, pharmacists are increasingly involved in therapy, medication monitoring, and dosing requirements, and it is prudent for them to become acquainted with the diagnostic imaging procedures used in medicine.

Some of these procedures do not involve ionizing radiation, but many do. X-ray emission is the most common type of ionizing radiation used, but other types such as beta and gamma may also be encountered.

This chapter examines the types of ionizing radiation that are commonly used in diagnostic imaging. The pharmacist with a basic understanding of the procedures and the radiations will be a more knowledgeable source for the medical team and will feel more comfortable reviewing and recommending medications for patients. In addition, the informed pharmacist will better understand the risks and benefits radiation presents to patients and clinicians.

First, it will be helpful to understand what ionizing radiation is and which of the various types of ionizing radiation a pharmacist may expect to encounter. This discussion will not include all the types of ionizing radiation but will focus instead on those pertinent to diagnostic imaging.

Parts of the Atom

We will briefly review the three main components of atoms: neutrons, protons, and electrons (Figure 2-1); we will refrain from discussing their subatomic components. Relating the particles and photons used in diagnostic imaging to neutrons, protons, and electrons will help the reader understand the basis for some of their actions and limitations in diagnostic imaging.

Any atom is composed of a positively charged center, the *nucleus,* and surrounding electrons that carry an opposing charge, balancing that of the nucleus. The electrons are constantly in motion around, but outside, the nucleus. In normal atoms, the number of electrons, each carrying a single negative charge, is equal to the number of protons, each carrying a single positive charge. Because these balance, the normal overall charge of an atom is neutral.

Neutrons and protons are jointly referred to as *nucleons.* The nucleons are of similar (but not the same) mass and are held together in the nucleus by a binding force referred to as the "strong interaction." Without the strong interaction to hold the nucleons together, the positively charged protons would not stay near each other and, though "buffered" by neutrons, would still repel each other.[1] For our purposes, we can state that different energy levels can be achieved within the nucleus, as well as induced energy imbalances due to changes in or

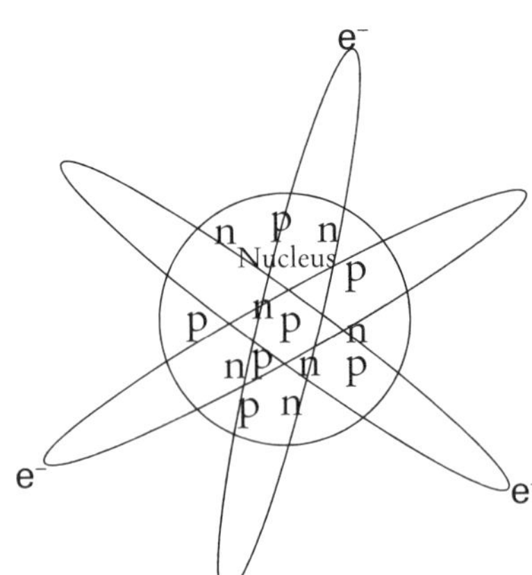

Figure 2-1. Simplified diagram of an atom, showing neutrons (n), protons (p), and electrons (e^-).

interactions with the nuclear particles. These times of imbalance are a root cause of photon and particle ejection from the nucleus.

Excitation, Ionization, and Pair Formation

Radiation is the release of energy by atoms in order to achieve a more energetically favorable (stable) state, with a lower potential energy. The energy released can be in the form of expelled particles or photons, depending on the mechanism the atom uses to send energy away (Figure 2-2). When the atom successfully releases this energy and thus becomes more stable, the effects of the emitted particles or photons ensue. Besides having value as the basis of diagnostic imaging, these emissions can interact with other, less desirable targets. The emissions may interact with matter in a harmless way, or in a way that causes damage or changes in DNA or other biologically important molecules (Figure 2-3). Thus, caution should be exercised during exposure to these emissions.[2,3] When certain types of radiation interact with atoms correctly, the radiation can cause excitation or ionization of the atoms and can possibly cause ion-pair formation.

Excitation occurs when some type of particle or photon strikes an electron, raising the electron to a higher potential energy orbital (shell). Normally, the electron then moves back to its original orbital and emits an x-ray to get rid of its extra energy (Figure 2-4). These x-rays can interact with tissues and DNA, as described below.

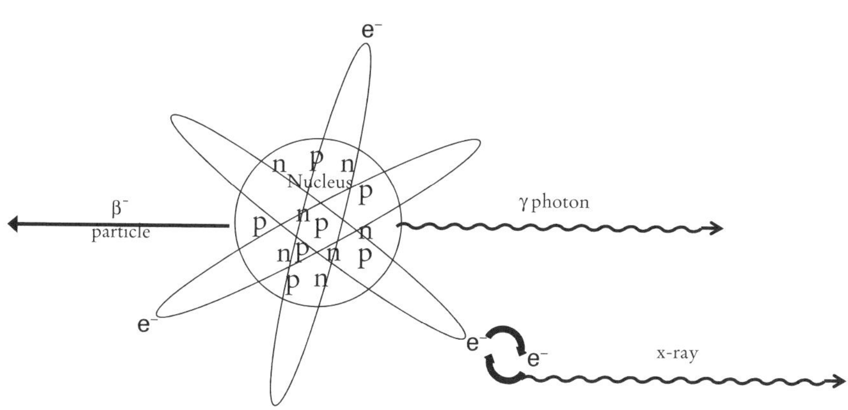

Figure 2-2. Mechanisms by which the atom can lose energy or particles.

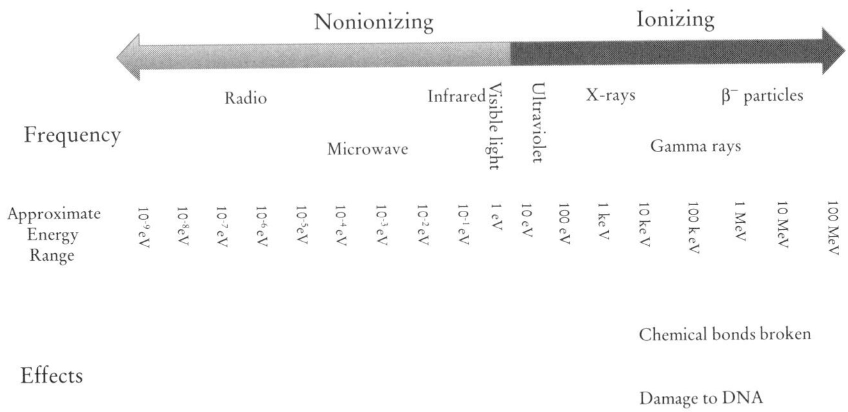

Figure 2-3. The right side of this continuum is the portion of the electromagnetic spectrum in which excitation, ionization, and pair formation can occur.

Ionization is the creation of positive or negative charges. Like excitation, ionization and pair formation occur when radiation interacts with orbital electrons. In this case, however, enough energy is imparted to one or more of these orbital electrons to completely dislodge them from their orbits and separate them from the atom. Thus, the atom, having lost one or more electrons, becomes posi-

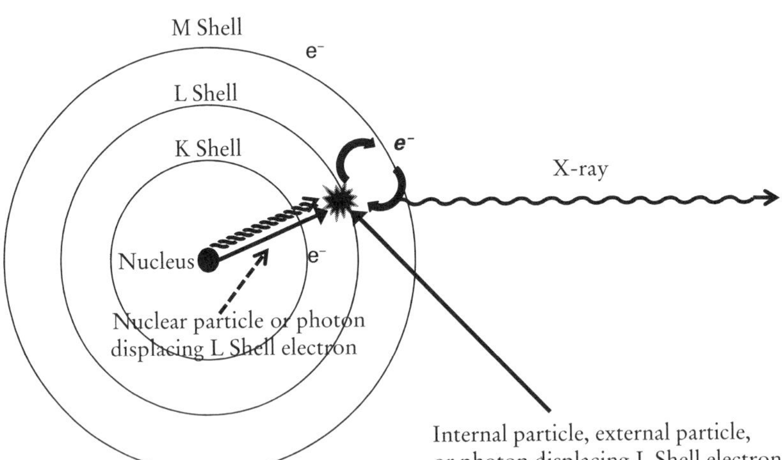

Figure 2-4. Excitation of orbital electrons by a nuclear emission, leading to x-ray emission. The L-shell electron temporarily occupies the M shell but falls back to the L shell, emitting an x-ray. The same mechanism occurs if the initiating radiation originates from outside the atom.

tively ionized. If the causative radiation is particulate (a particle), a neighboring atom or molecule also may be ionized by the interaction, gaining the electron(s) and becoming negatively charged. This phenomenon is called *ion-pair formation.* If the particle is charged to begin with (an alpha or beta particle, discussed later), the ionizations can be induced not only by physical interaction with orbital electrons but also by charge interactions (attraction, repulsion) with the electrons of neighboring atoms. Ions can proceed to interact with tissues and DNA, as described below.

Ionization (ejection of an orbital electron) can occur with as little energy input as 34 electron volts (eV). Electromagnetic photons are considered to be ionizing if their energy exceeds 124 eV. Excitation often requires even less energy than ionization.

Photons and Particles

Physicists would point out that there is little to differentiate between a photon and a particle, because their wave and particle characteristics are interchangeable. For our purposes, however, we will define a *photon* as an electromagnetic emission (from inside or outside the nucleus) having a defined *wavelength* but no mass, whereas a *particle* has a defined mass and carries a *charge,* positive or negative, sometimes having a magnitude greater than 1.

Electrons orbit the nucleus at defined energy levels. Those electrons closer to the nucleus possess higher *kinetic* energy (lower *potential* energy), and those farther away, lower kinetic energy. Although the orbits of electrons around the nucleus are not neat, concentric circles, they can be visualized as such in order to illustrate energy changes that occur when electrons move between orbitals or out of orbitals. Figure 2-5 conceptualizes a "generic" atom, with a core of nucleons surrounded by the electron orbital energy levels K, L, and M. If an electron moves in, toward the nucleus, such as from L to K, it loses potential energy. This lost energy cannot simply disappear. It is released as an x-ray, which leaves the vicinity of the atom.

Emissions that are of interest in diagnostic imaging include the particles β^+ and β^- originating from the nucleus, gamma (γ) photons originating from the nucleus, and x-rays originating from the electron movements between orbitals.

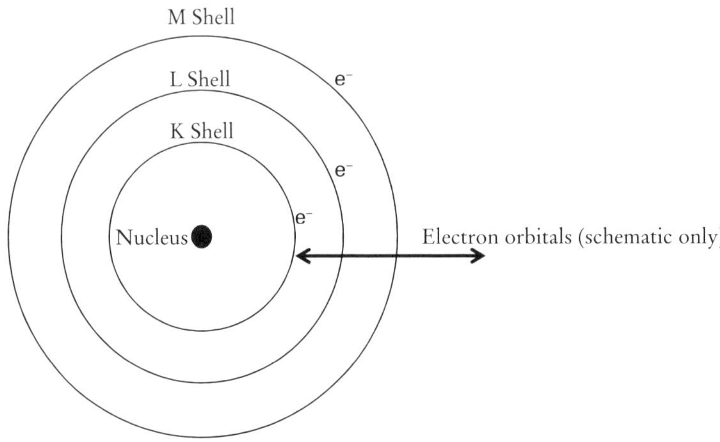

Figure 2-5. A "generic" atom, with a core of nucleons surrounded by electrons in the orbital energy levels K, L, and M.

Energy Expressions

Particles and photons can be assigned energy values by using the equation $E = mc^2$. In this equation E is energy, expressed in ergs (grams·cm²/sec²), but is interconvertible with mass (m, in grams), and c is the value for the speed of light (2.997925×10^{10} cm/sec).[4] Knowing the energy valuation for particles and photons is important, because it is the energy of particles and photons that is the basis for their use in imaging.

The Units keV and MeV

Although the use of ergs to express emission energies is legitimate, in practice the use of electron volts (eV) is the rule. A volt is a common unit of potential. An electron volt is a unit of energy. An eV is the equivalent of 1.6×10^{-12} ergs. The energies involved in diagnostic imaging are quite a bit larger: thousands (kilo) and millions (mega) of electron volts, written keV and MeV, respectively; 1 keV equals 1000 eV and 1 MeV equals 1000 keV. For use in diagnostic imaging there are various energy optima for best performance and detection, depending on the procedure. The energies of x-rays, γ photons, and β^- particles are compared in Figure 2-6.

The emission energies are used, or created (in the case of x-rays), for their favorable imaging properties. Although photons (i.e., x-rays

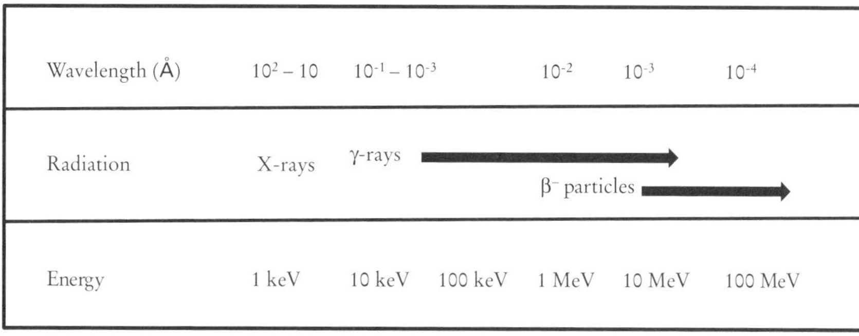

Figure 2-6. Photons and particles have different properties that endow each with its unique usefulness in diagnostic imaging. Shorter wavelength implies higher energy.

and γ-rays) have energy, they are massless and have no associated charge. They therefore are less able to cause excitation, ionization, and pair production than are particles. They also tend to be monoenergetic (of one wavelength/emission energy), which improves imaging quality.

Effects of Excitation, Ionization, and Pair Formation

Some radiation itself can cause ionization. When it is capable of doing so, it is called "ionizing radiation." Since many radiations carry energies in the MeV range, it is not surprising that ions can be created from radiation. Breaking a carbon–carbon double bond requires only 4.9 eV, and ionization requires as little as 34 eV. So, breaking covalent bonds and creating ions from ionizing radiation can occur quite easily.

Free radicals can also result from radiation interactions. Free radicals are chemically very reactive and can damage tissues and DNA. Damage to DNA can cause cell death, mutations, or carcinogenesis.

Free radical formation from water takes place through the following reactions:

$$H_2O \rightarrow H_2O^+ + e^-$$

$$H_2O^+ \rightarrow H_2O \rightarrow H_3O^+ + OH^\bullet \text{ (free radical, very chemically reactive)}$$

Electromagnetic photons (x-rays and γ-rays) are considered ionizing if their energy exceeds approximately 124 eV, which is a level consistent with all diagnostic imaging x-rays and γ-rays.

Electromagnetic radiation is considered to be indirectly ionizing, whereas particulate radiation (β^-, an electron ejected from the nucleus; more about these later), because of its original charge, is considered to be *directly* ionizing. β^- particles can dislodge orbital electrons or attract positively charged entities. Both directly ionizing and indirectly ionizing radiation can damage tissue or DNA or create free radicals.

Ionizing Radiation Used for Diagnostic Imaging

Radiations used for diagnostic imaging have different energies, may be particles or photons, and are useful in different procedures. All of these types of radiation are capable of ionization, excitation, and pair formation.

X-Rays

X-rays used for diagnostic imaging are man-made, external radiation. X-rays are produced when an electron is given energy (usually by an incoming radiation, particle, or photon) that causes the temporary occupation by the electron of a higher potential energy orbital (i.e., farther from the nucleus). To get rid of this acquired energy the displaced electrons fall back toward the nucleus and return to their original orbitals. To do so the electrons must give off kinetic energy in the form of x-rays. This is illustrated in Figure 2-4, where a nuclear or extranuclear particle or photon strikes an L-shell orbital electron, temporarily raising it to the M shell, with subsequent release of energy in the form of an x-ray as the electron returns to the L shell.

Since the change in energy associated with an orbital move is a defined and invariable quantity for a particular move, the resulting emitted x-rays are usually *monoenergetic* (meaning "same energy"). By design, they have the energy desired for optimum imaging for the given procedure (such as standard "x-rays," computed tomography [CT], fluoroscopy, or mammography).

Bombardment of materials ideal for the type of interaction desired produces x-ray energies most favorable for the procedure being performed (Figure 2-7). Generally, these x-ray energies are designed to fall between 20 and 150 keV (relatively low-energy photons), based on whatever energy optimizes the imaging procedure. Because they are photon emissions, x-rays can be assigned wavelengths. The details of this are beyond the scope of this chapter.

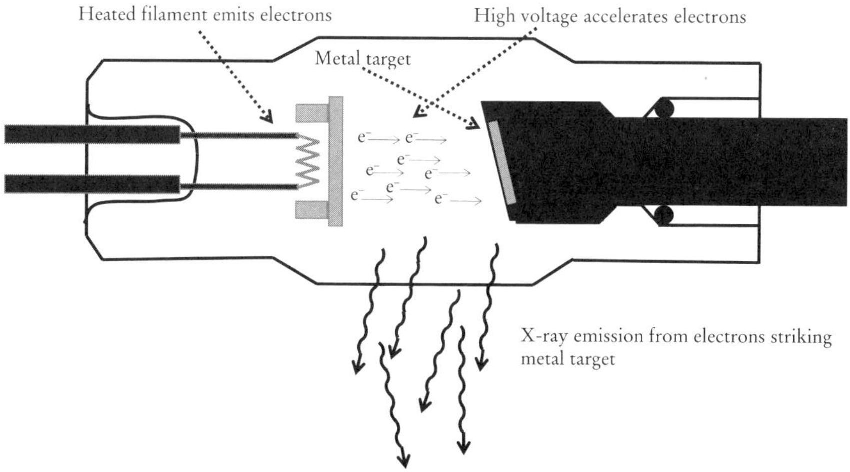

Figure 2-7. Artificial production of x-rays for use in diagnostic imaging.

The x-rays produced are directed at the area of the body being studied. X-rays are used for their ability to cause exposure of x-ray films or other, more modern collection devices. Their usefulness lies in the differing absorption characteristics of different types of body tissues.[5] The densities of various tissues cause them to absorb x-rays differently, thus transmitting different quantities of photons onto the x-ray film or capturing device and enabling an image to be produced. Depending on the energy of the x-ray, more or fewer of the photons will be absorbed by soft tissue or more dense tissue, allowing clinicians to visualize and diagnose diseases (e.g., in mammography).

Gamma (γ) Radiation

Gamma rays also are photons (nonparticulate), but they originate in the nucleus (Figure 2-8). They are emitted to relieve excess nuclear excitation energy. Since they are photons, gammas have no charge. Like x-rays, they are electromagnetic radiation moving at the speed of light. Gamma photons are monoenergetic, with the exact energy dependent upon the isotope of origin. Being monoenergetic makes them very useful for imaging in nuclear medicine. Gamma photons range from 1 keV to 10 MeV (generally higher than the range for x-rays) but are most useful for diagnostic imaging when between 100 and 200 keV. Gamma photons are used for diagnostic imaging when radioactive isotopes are

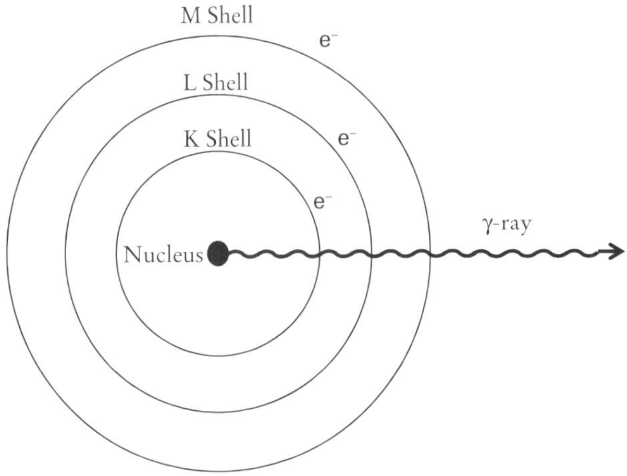

Figure 2-8. Gamma photons are emitted from the nucleus as a result of energy changes within the nucleus.

placed inside the body. Gamma detection falls under the purview of nuclear medicine. Images are collected by using the abilities of certain crystals to scintillate (flash) upon exposure to γ-rays. Thus, γ-photon procedures can be conceptualized as "x-rays from the inside out." With γ-rays, unlike x-rays, the criterion for obtaining valuable images is not always varied attenuation; instead, information pertaining to the location, movement, and physiology of a disease can be acquired.

Beta (β^-) Emissions

β^- ("beta minus") emissions are negatively charged particles expelled from the nucleus; they can be conceptualized as highly energetic electrons (Figure 2-9). Like electrons, β^- particles carry a negative charge. However, they are not orbital electrons but are ejected particles that originate in the nucleus. β^- particles are expelled at high velocity and therefore have intrinsic kinetic energy in addition to their negative charge. β^- particles are assigned energies according to experimental data from known β^- emitters. For a given type of nuclear interaction, a certain range of β^- energies is expelled.[6] Within this range of energies, maximum and average energies can be measured, thus identifying the isotope of origin through comparison with known standards (Figure 2-10).[7]

β^- particles can be used for imaging purposes, although the image quality is lower than that obtained with other imaging modalities. This

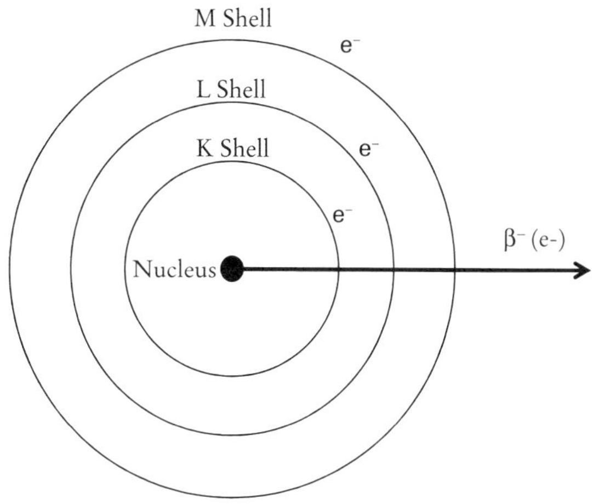

Figure 2-9. Beta (β^-) particles are emitted from within the nucleus as a result of energy changes within the nucleus.

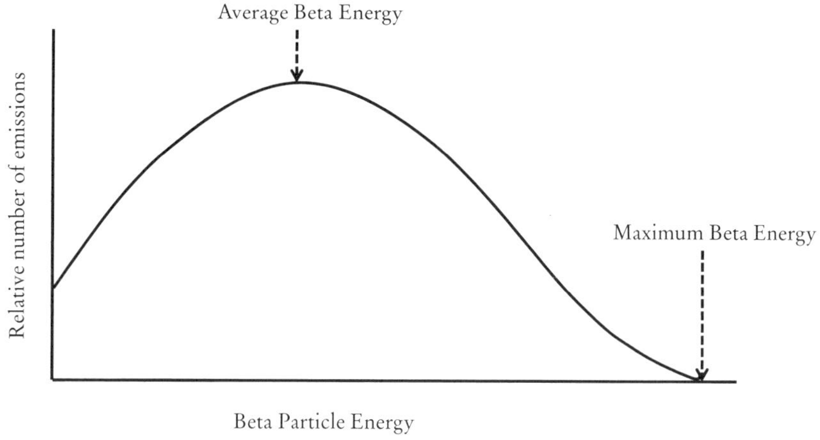

Figure 2-10. Beta (and positron) particles have a spectrum of energy of emission for a particular type of emission. The energy curve produced can be used for identifying the source or deciding if the emission has the proper characteristics to be useful.

is because β^- particles, instead of being monoenergetic, have a range of energies and because their relatively high energies (often from 200 keV up to the MeV range) make it difficult for equipment to collect emissions and produce high-quality diagnostic images. β^- particles may be classified as "soft" (under 200 keV) or "hard" (200–300 keV or higher). Being charged, high intrinsic energy particles, β^- particles are relatively efficient at creating ionization, pair production, and free radicals.

β^- particles often find use in therapeutic applications because of their ability to cause ionization and pair production. This is essential for the tissue and DNA destruction commonly used in such procedures as cancer treatment.

Positrons (β^+)

β^+ (positron) emissions are also particles expelled from the nucleus, but these can be conceptualized as positively charged electrons. They are called *positrons* and carry a "positive 1" (1+) charge. Unlike β^- particles, positrons are not long-lived; they interact with environmental electrons soon after leaving the nucleus. During this interaction, termed *annihilation,* the positive and negative charges cancel each other. Annihilation is not without energy balance. The annihilation results in the ejection of two photons of equal energy (511 keV) at nearly 180° to each other (Figure 2-11).

Like β^- emissions, β^+ particles result from changes within the nucleus. β^+ particles are ejected from the nucleus at a high velocity but over a range of energies. Unlike β^- particles, the energy positrons carry is unimportant. It is their reaction with electrons, producing two 511-keV γ photons that propagate 180° relative to each other, that is the key property for imaging purposes. The annihilation photons and their monoenergetic nature are the basis for positron emission tomography (PET) and the exquisite images obtainable with this technology. Although positrons themselves are charged particles, the conversion to photons decreases their ability to induce ionization, pair production, and free radicals.

Alpha (α^{2+}) Emission

Although it is not used for diagnostic imaging, α^{2+} emission is briefly described here because it was previously mentioned as an ionizing,

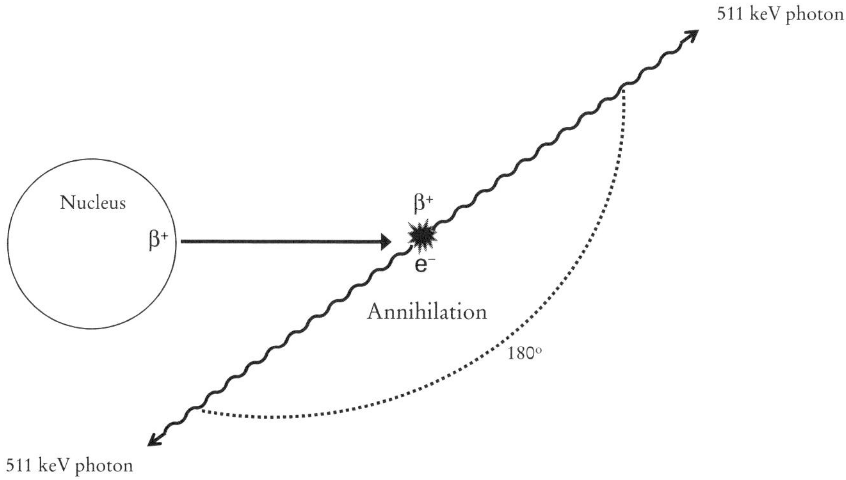

Figure 2-11. Emission of a positron and annihilation from its interaction with an electron. Positrons (positively charged β particles) originate in the nucleus from energy changes within the nucleus. They quickly encounter an environmental electron, annihilate, and release two 511-keV photons, directed 180° from each other.

and thus potentially pair-forming, radioactive emission. An alpha particle is a helium nucleus with both electrons missing. Therefore, it carries a net "positive 2" (2+) charge.[8] Because it is a large particle and is doubly ionized, it has potential for extreme damage to cellular components such as DNA.

Summary

Many, though not all, diagnostic imaging procedures employ some type of ionizing radiation. This radiation may be from an external source (x-rays) or from internal sources (gamma, beta, and positron [annihilation photons]). Ionizing radiation can be electromagnetic (photon) or particulate, although the distinction between the two types can be imprecise. X-rays are created to fit a desired energy for the procedure involved. Gamma photons and beta particles have energies particular to the radioisotope of origin, or energy of production. Positrons produce particular and predictable photon energy. Procedures that use these are designed to be optimized for the energy of emission.

References

1. Georgia State University. Fundamental forces. 2008. http://hyperphysics.phy-astr.gsu.edu/hbase/forces/funfor.html. Accessed January 23, 2011.
2. International Commission on Radiological Protection. Publication 26: Recommendations of the International Commission on Radiological Protection. New York: Pergamon; 1978.
3. International Commission on Radiological Protection. Publication 60: Recommendations of the International Commission on Radiological Protection (*Annals of the International Commission on Radiological Protection.* Vol 21:1–3). New York: Elsevier; 1990.
4. Georgia State University. Fundamental physical constants. 2008. http://hyperphysics.phy-astr.gsu.edu/hbase/tables/funcon.html. Accessed January 23, 2011.
5. Lawson RS. Introduction to radioactivity. 1999. www.e-radiography.net/articles/Introduction%20to%20Radioactivity.pdf. Accessed August 5, 2011.
6. Kurie FND, Richardson JR, Paxton HC. The radiations emitted from artificially produced radioactive substances. I. The upper limits and shapes of the β-ray spectra from several elements. *Phys Rev.* 1936;49:368–81.
7. Loevinger R. Average energy of allowed beta-particle spectra. *Phys Med Biol.* 1957;1:330–9.
8. Holloway MG, Livingston MS. Range and specific ionization of alpha-particles. *Phys Rev.* 1938;54:18–37.

Further Reading and Web Sources

Clarke FW, Thorpe TE, Seubert K. Report of the International Commission on Atomic Weights. *J Am Chem Soc.* 1903;25:1–5.

Hall E. *Radiobiology for the Radiobiologist.* Philadelphia: Lippincott Williams & Wilkins; 2000.

Idaho State University. Radiation Information Network's radiation-related terms. www.physics.isu.edu/radinf/terms.htm. Accessed January 23, 2011.

Japan Atomic Energy Agency. Chart of the nuclides 2010. wwwndc.jaea.go.jp/CN10/CNALL.html#root. Accessed August 5, 2011.

Kowalsky RJ, Falen SW, eds. *Radiopharmaceuticals in Nuclear Pharmacy and Nuclear Medicine.* 3rd ed. Washington, DC: American Pharmacists Association; 2011.

Los Alamos National Laboratory. Periodic table of the elements. http://periodic.lanl.gov/43.shtml. Accessed January 23, 2011.

Mattauch J. The rational choice of a unified scale for atomic weights and nuclidic masses. Supplement to E. Wichers Report on Atomic Weights for 1956–57. *J Am Chem Soc.* 1958;80:4121.

Nucleonica. Decay schemes. www.nucleonica.net/Applet/Decay/radioactive_decay.aspx. Accessed August 5, 2011.

Princeton University. Radiation Safety Guide. Appendix E: Roentgens, RADs, REMs, and other units. http://web.princeton.edu/sites/ehs/radsafeguide/rsg_app_e.htm. Accessed January 23, 2011.

Saha G. *Fundamentals of Nuclear Pharmacy.* New York: Springer; 2004.

Wang CH, Willis DL, Loveland WD. *Radiotracer Methodology in the Biological, Environmental, and Physical Sciences.* Englewood Cliffs, NJ: Prentice-Hall; 1975.

CHAPTER 3

Review of Imaging Procedures Using X-Rays

Cory Duncan

A goal of the field of medicine is to understand the structure and function of the human body and how it is affected by health, illness, and injury. With the discovery of x-rays and the radiograph, the discipline of radiology was born and immediately became a powerful force in the diagnosis and treatment of disease. Advances in medical imaging over the past century have paralleled society's growth in the fields of science, technology, and computing. The first radiographs processed more than 100 years ago were of poor quality by today's standards and took as long as one-half hour to capture. Today, cross-sectional images of the entire human body can be obtained and reconstructed into detailed three-dimensional images within minutes.[1]

Prior to the discovery of the radiograph, physicians were limited in their ability to obtain information about the human body, health, and illness. They truly practiced the "art of medicine" and were guided by their experience, their knowledge, and their five senses. Wilhelm Roentgen's discovery of x-rays and production of the radiograph provided a window into the human body through which physicians and health care providers could further advance the mission of medicine.

History

Wilhelm Conrad Roentgen discovered x-rays in 1895 while experimenting with cathode tubes in his laboratory at the University of Würzburg, Germany. Roentgen was studying the effects of cathode light emissions on screens composed of barium platinocyanide that fluoresce when exposed to ultraviolet light from energized cathodes. On November 8, 1895, Roentgen encased a cathode in a light-tight cardboard wrapping. When he energized the cathode, a screen lying on a nearby laboratory bench began to fluoresce. Roentgen realized that a new type of energy was escaping the enclosed cathode, a "light that never was."[2] This energy, invisible to the naked eye, penetrated substances that would block visible light. Roentgen named these new rays after the algebraic unknown, *x*, and the term "x-ray" was born.

Roentgen confined himself to his laboratory, testing a variety of substances for their ability to block x-rays. He quickly learned that x-rays could penetrate various materials and could be recorded on photographic plates. When Roentgen's wife became suspicious of his new, time-consuming research, he invited her to witness this new discovery. On December 22, 1895, Roentgen produced the first known human radiograph—of his wife's hand.[3]

Roentgen published his revolutionary work on December 28, 1895, in the University of Würzburg's *Proceedings of the Physical–Medical Society.* His discovery of x-rays captivated the world of science, and in 1896 alone over 1000 articles pertaining to x-rays were published in journals around the world.[2] In this chapter, we will discuss three major radiologic imaging modalities that utilize the x-rays Roentgen discovered: radiography, computed tomography (CT), and fluoroscopy.

X-Rays

X-rays are electromagnetic radiation composed of photons. The electromagnetic spectrum begins with the very long wavelength radio waves used in magnetic resonance imaging (MRI). As the wavelengths shorten, the spectrum proceeds through microwaves, infrared light, visible light, ultraviolet light, and x-rays and terminates with the short-wavelength gamma rays used in nuclear imaging.[4]

X-rays used in radiographic procedures are produced in *x-ray tubes.* X-ray tubes are airtight vacuums containing two electrodes: a cathode and an anode (Figure 3-1). A metal (usually tungsten) filament

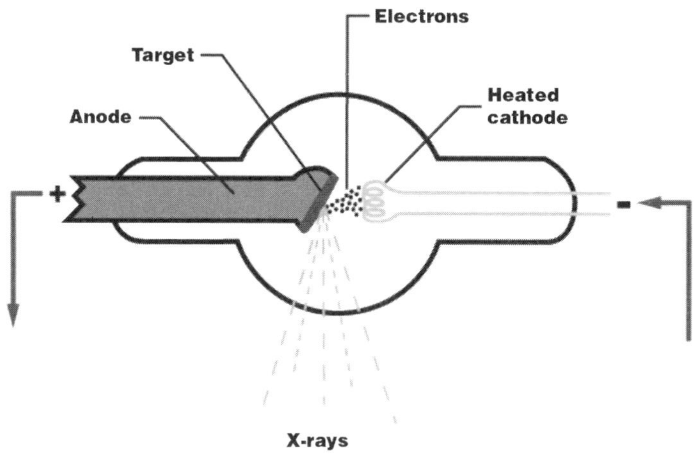

Figure 3-1. Basic x-ray tube. (Image courtesy of Kara Weatherman.)

with a high melting point within the cathode assembly is subjected to an electric current, much as in a light bulb. This process, by thermal excitation, liberates electrons that travel toward the anode. A portion of the energy released when electrons strike the anode is in the form of x-rays.[1] All three imaging modalities discussed in this chapter (plain film radiography, CT, and fluoroscopy) employ this basic concept of x-ray generation in their respective imaging chains.

Radiography

The generation of x-rays within the x-ray tube is the first step in the radiographic imaging sequence. Next, x-rays are directed through an aluminum filter that absorbs low-energy x-rays that are useless in standard imaging processes and would deliver unnecessary radiation to the patient. High-energy x-rays pass through the filter and are directed through a radiopaque collimator that shapes the x-ray beam and minimizes the scatter of x-rays. The collimator can be adjusted to create a window of x-ray energy that is the appropriate size for the desired radiograph and limits the body area to be irradiated.[4]

Traditional radiographs are produced when x-rays contact a cassette containing radiographic film. The film is surrounded on both sides by screens that fluoresce when struck by x-rays. The film within the cassette is exposed directly by the interaction with x-rays, but it is exposed to a greater extent by the fluorescence of the adjacent screens.[5]

The inclusion of fluorescent screens allows a smaller amount of x-rays to be used, limiting the patient's radiation exposure.

Digital radiographs are standard in most radiology departments today. Digital cassettes capture images on reusable *storage phosphors.* When exposed to laser light, phosphors release their stored information to an image processor that converts the energy into a digital image. This process has an advantage over traditional film exposure because it requires smaller doses of radiation for image processing. Computer postprocessing allows digital radiographs to be enhanced, whereas traditional images cannot be manipulated after exposure of the film. A major advantage of digital images is their ability to be easily stored, transported, and archived. *Picture archiving and communication systems* (PACS), present in most hospitals and health care systems, allow medical images to be transferred and viewed immediately throughout hospital information networks along with other patient information.

Conventional radiograph machines (Figure 3-2) are commonplace in most physician offices, urgent care centers, emergency departments, and hospitals. Larger medical establishments often have multiple machines specially designed for imaging various body parts.

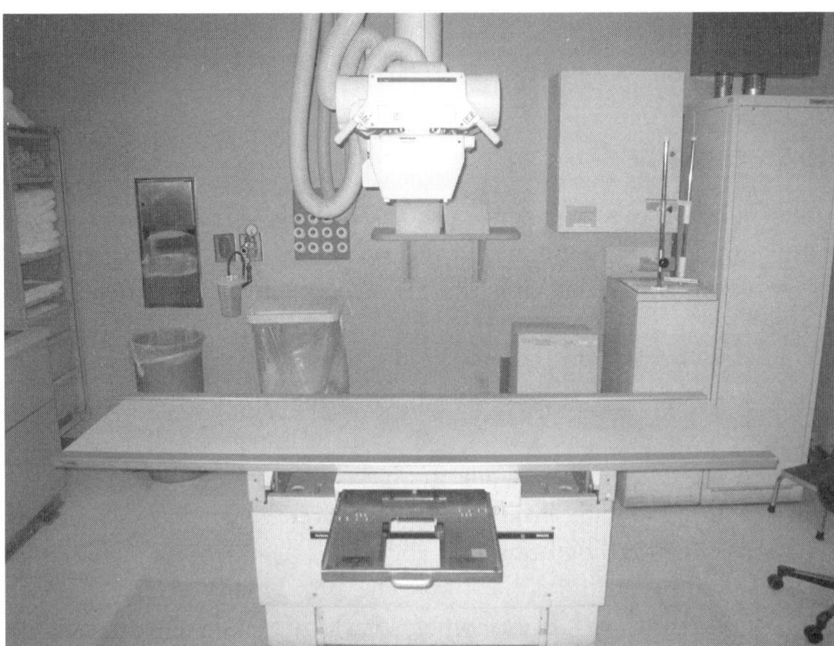

Figure 3-2. Standard radiograph equipment. (Image courtesy of Cory Duncan.)

Radiographs are viewed in shades of black, gray, and white. As x-rays travel through matter they are absorbed, attenuated, and scattered. The degree of these interactions is related to the density of the object through which they pass.[5] X-rays pass through entirely radiolucent objects with little to no disruption, and when they contact radiographic film a black image is produced. Conversely, x-rays are unable to pass through radiopaque objects, and the receiving film is left unexposed and white. Between these two extremes of exposure are shades of gray that are produced by variable x-ray absorption and attenuation related to object density.

Within the human body there are five basic substances with which x-rays interact: air, fat, water, bone, and metals (Figure 3-3). Air is completely radiolucent and appears black on radiographs. Fat (adipose tissue) has a density slightly greater than that of air and appears nearly black. Muscles, organs, and other soft tissues appear in a range of gray colors between black and white depending on the structure's water content and tissue density. Objects containing high concentrations of calcium (teeth, bones, and calcified tumors) absorb most of the x-rays passing through them and appear in varying shades of white on radiographs. Intravenous contrast agents, most surgical hardware, bullets, ingested coins, batteries, and other metal foreign bodies will block all x-rays and appear bright white (Figure 3-4).

Interpretation of radiographic films requires a firm understanding of three-dimensional human anatomy and the ability to visualize it inside a two-dimensional image. In a single radiographic view, x-rays travel through multiple body tissues of varying density. For example, in a radiograph of the chest, as x-rays travel through the midline of the

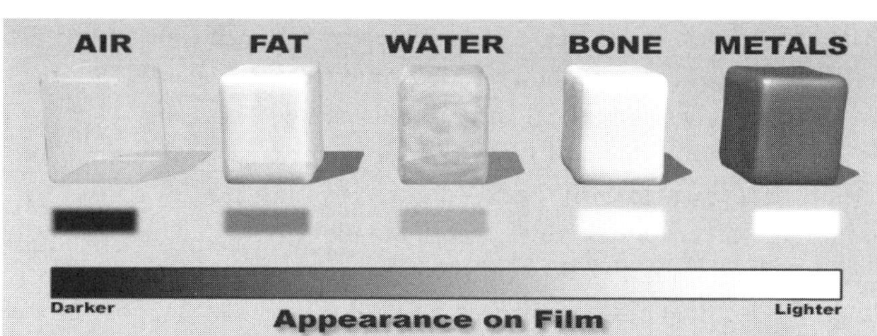

Figure 3-3. Interaction of x-rays with various human tissues. (Image courtesy of Kara Weatherman.)

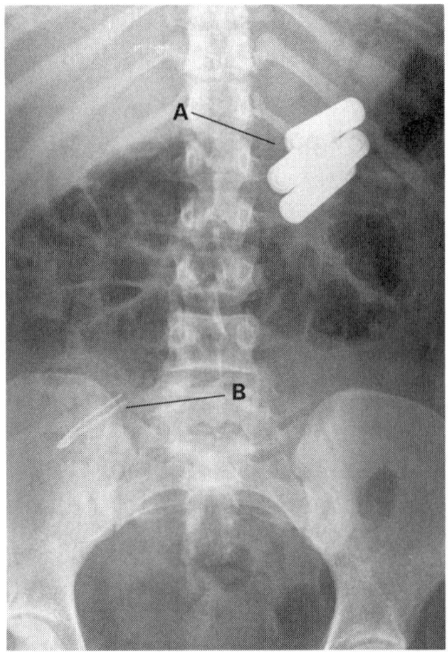

Figure 3-4. Abdominal radiograph showing two types of radiodense foreign bodies: (A) a collection of batteries and (B) a folded wire from an eyeglass frame. (Image courtesy of Cory Duncan.)

thorax they encounter the bony sternum, the heart, large blood vessels within the mediastinum, the esophagus, and the spine before striking and exposing the two-dimensional radiographic film (Figure 3-5A). The resultant exposure on the radiograph will be from the cumulative absorption, attenuation, and scatter the x-rays encounter through that plane of the body. Obtaining diagnostic information from a single view of a body part when multiple tissues overlap can fail to reveal concealed pathology and is inadequate (Figure 3-5B). Multiple images are usually taken of the same body part from different angles, or perspectives, commonly from lateral and oblique views.

Throughout the body, radiographs are used to diagnose and classify fractures of bones and identify foreign bodies in the soft tissues. Chest radiographs are essential in identifying pneumonia, pulmonary edema, masses, and other space-occupying processes in the lungs. Abdominal radiographs can be used to quickly diagnose bowel obstructions or perforations.

Radiographs are the most common imaging modality used by clinicians and are the first-line imaging modality for the evaluation

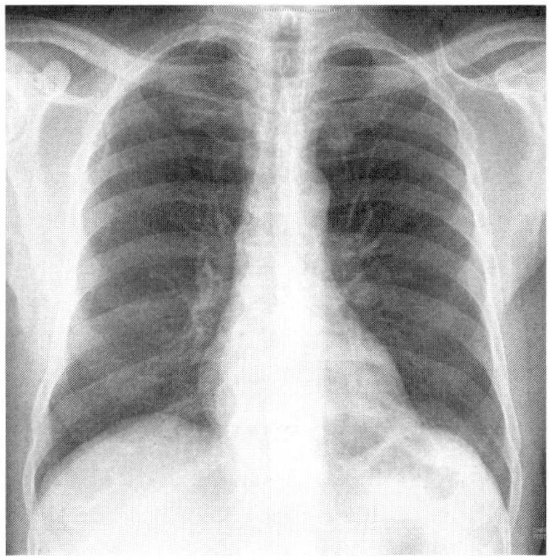

Figure 3-5A. Anterior–posterior (AP) chest radiograph of a patient presenting with fever and cough. The lung fields are clear. (Image courtesy of Cory Duncan.)

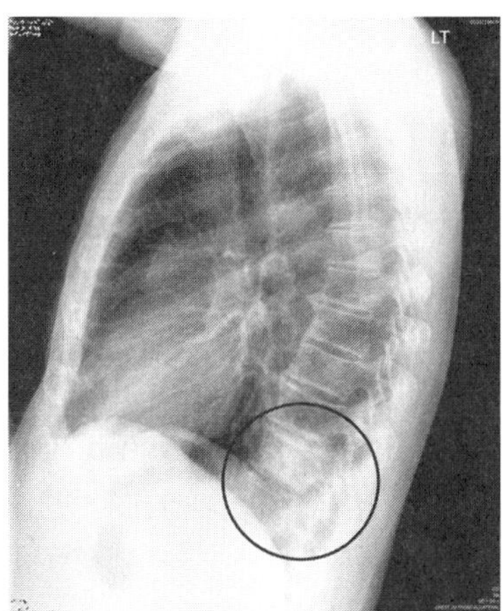

Figure 3-5B. Lateral radiograph of patient in Figure 3-5A, showing a dense consolidation in the lower lobe indicated by the circled area. This finding is consistent with pneumonia and emphasizes the importance of multiple views. On the AP view, the infiltrate is hidden behind the heart and diaphragm. (Image courtesy of Cory Duncan.)

of abnormal health and the diagnosis and screening of most medical illnesses and injuries. Radiographic images are obtained and processed rapidly, can be acquired outside the radiology department with portable equipment, use very low doses of radiation compared with other imaging modalities, and reveal well-known patterns of health and disease that can be interpreted quickly by most clinicians.

Mammography

Mammography is a special form of plain film radiography that uses low-energy x-rays (blocked in other radiographic techniques by filtering) to capture images of the human breast. Breast tissue is composed of fat, glandular tissue, and other soft tissues that make tissue differentiation difficult with standard plain radiograph techniques. Low-energy x-rays accentuate subtle differences in breast tissue. Mammography is used to evaluate suspected or known breast disease in both males and females and can detect breast carcinomas in early stages when they are only millimeters in size. The goal of mammography is to detect breast carcinomas (masses and microcalcifications) as early as possible before they become palpable or symptomatic or have the opportunity to metastasize (Figure 3-6).

Mammography is performed in machines specially designed to accommodate the human breast. *Screening mammography* is performed on normal, asymptomatic patients at routine intervals under recommended guidelines, with the intent of identifying breast carcinomas as early as possible. Screening mammograms include two images of each breast, a mediolateral oblique (MLO) view and a craniocaudal (CC) view. *Diagnostic mammography* is performed if an abnormality is identified on screening images or if there are symptoms suspicious of breast carcinoma (overlying skin changes, palpable mass, nipple discharge). Diagnostic images are more complex than screening images and utilize many different views according to patient-specific issues. Magnification compression views are used to further evaluate microcalcifications, and spot compression views are obtained when concerning masses or focal asymmetries are seen in screening images.

Mammography is an excellent tool for the screening and diagnosis of breast carcinomas when coupled with routine breast self-evaluations. The diagnosis and treatment of breast disorders does not end with mammography alone. When breast abnormalities (both benign and malig-

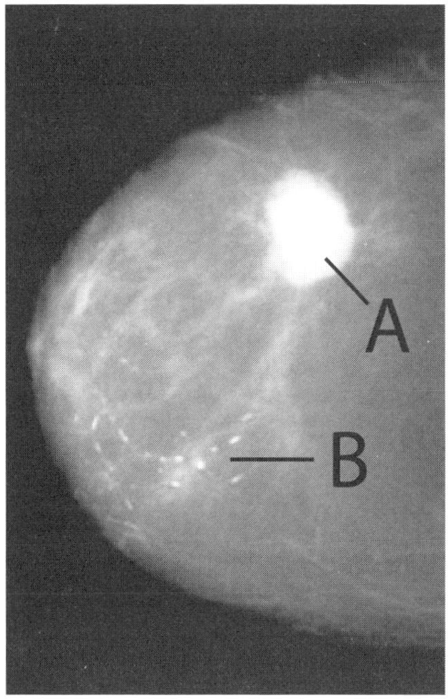

Figure 3-6. Mammograph showing a large dense mass (A) and microcalcifications (B). (Image courtesy of Kara Weatherman.)

nant) are discovered, mammography is often coupled with ultrasound (US), MRI, and interventional techniques to comprehensively manage breast disease.

Fluoroscopy

Fluoroscopy is a form of radiologic imaging that uses the principles of x-ray generation; however, image output is in the form of a "video x-ray." During a fluoroscopic exam, continuous or pulsating beams of x-rays are directed at an organ or body part of interest. Instead of exposing a radiographic film, x-rays strike an image intensifier that increases the brightness of the image and converts it to a video signal that can be viewed on a monitor and converted to digital images. Fluoroscopic images generally show contrast opposite that of traditional radiographs; air and radiolucent substances appear white, soft tissues are seen in shades of gray depending on density, and radiopaque items are black.

Fluoroscopy is widely used in interventional radiology suites and operating rooms where immediate, real-time information is required for medical or surgical procedures. Not only can fluoroscopy be used to provide diagnostic information in relevant areas, but it can assist and guide therapeutic procedures as well. In interventional radiology, fluoroscopy relies on the use of endoluminal contrast agents to provide real-time information on the patency of blood vessels. The injection of focal doses of contrast through catheters inserted into blood vessels and observation of the movement of contrast into and out of the area of interest assists in the diagnosis of arterial occlusion, thrombosis, hemorrhage, and aneurysm (Figures 3-7A through 3-7E). Knowledge of vessel patency and dynamics is integral in the placement of deep-vein thrombosis filters, arterial stents, and aneurysmal clips and coils.

Gastrointestinal contrast agents (oral and rectal) are given to patients undergoing fluoroscopic evaluation of the esophagus, stomach, intestines, and rectum to evaluate motility, patency, and anatomy. Contrast can be introduced into the reproductive and urinary systems for evaluation under fluoroscopy. Orthopedic procedures rely heavily on fluoroscopy in the operating room to assist in the alignment and fixation of broken bones, the placement of artificial joints, and the application of other orthopedic hardware.

Computed Tomography

X-ray *computed tomography* (CT), also referred to as *computed axial tomography* (CAT), is an imaging modality that produces cross-sectional images of the human body based on the x-ray attenuation properties of the tissues being imaged. Godfrey N. Hounsfield developed the first CT scanner in 1972, based on research by Allan M. Cormack. In 1979 the two men were awarded the Nobel Prize in Physiology or Medicine for their work. Hounsfield and Cormack's machine was dedicated to imaging of the head, and in 1974 Robert S. Ledley developed the first whole-body CT scanner. The development of the CT scanner revolutionized the field of medicine and changed the way clinicians practiced in a way that no other technology has. It can be argued that CT technology has been the most significant contribution to the field of medicine in the past 40 years.

In CT machines, x-rays are produced by x-ray tubes, interact with the patient, and are measured by an x-ray detector. The x-ray tube gantry of the CT scanner has a large circular opening in the center through which the patient couch passes and the x-ray tube/detector assembly

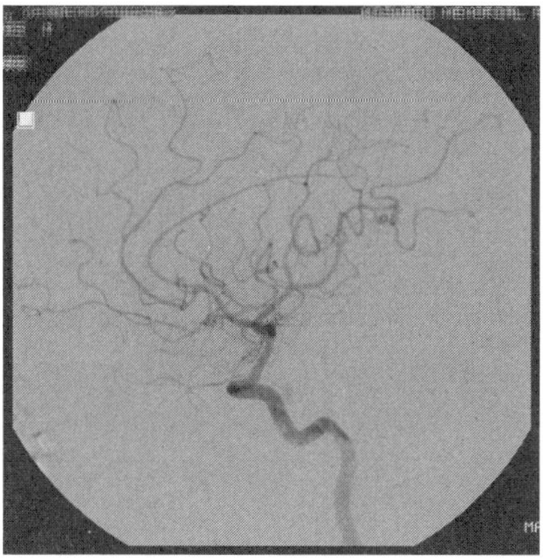

A

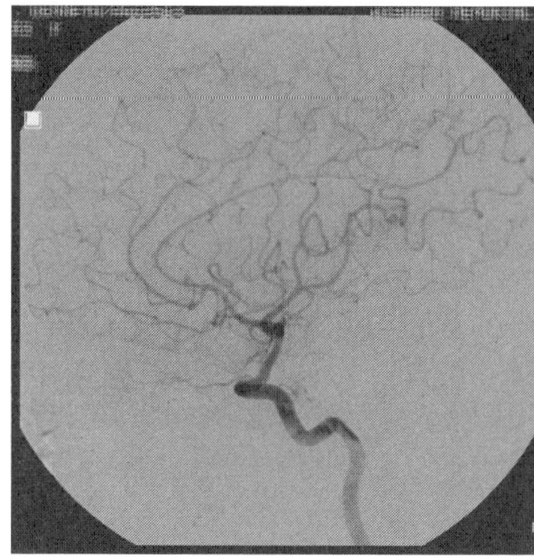

B

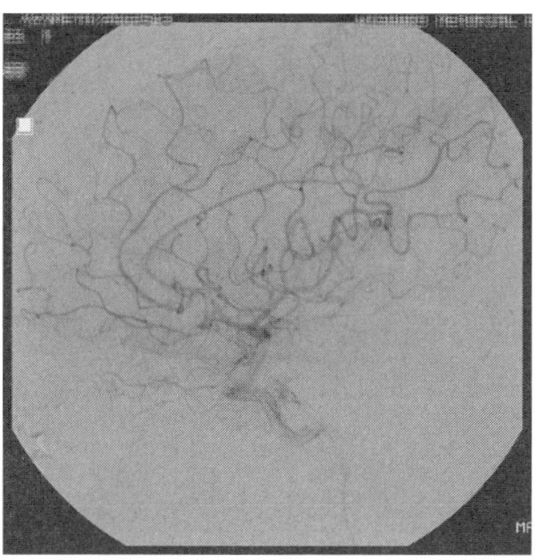

C

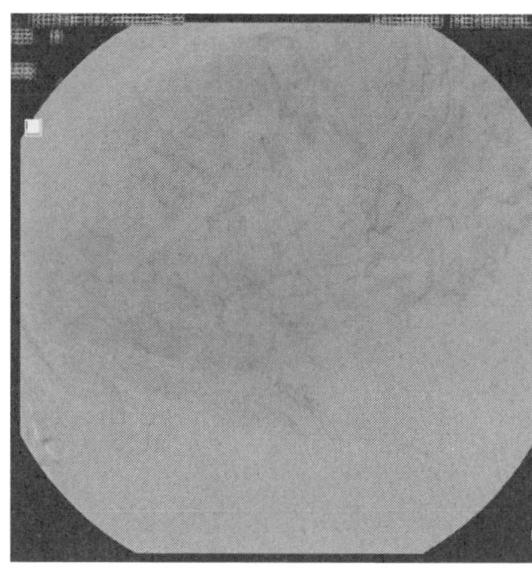

D

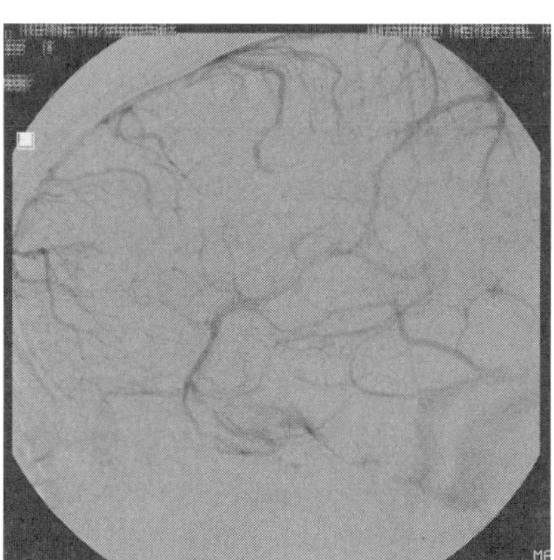

E

Figure 3-7. Selected sequential images of intravenous contrast moving through cerebral vasculature during angiography. Images show contrast moving through the arterial vessels (A–C), blood pooling in small vessels and capillaries (D), and finally movement of contrast into venous vasculature (E). (Images courtesy of Cory Duncan.)

rotates (Figure 3-8). A computer controls the couch as it passes through the gantry in specific increments (1–10 mm) depending on the indications for the study and the specific area of the body imaged.

For each slice of the body, the x-ray tube/detector assembly rotates 360° around the patient. A fan of x-ray beams is transmitted through the body and measured by the detector 180° from the x-ray tube (Figure 3-9). During each rotation, multiple tissue-attenuation measurements are obtained from all possible angles and all possible distances from the center. On the basis of all of the measurements in one rotation, the actual attenuation at each point is known and can be used to reconstruct a cross-sectional image at that level.

Traditional CT images are obtained and viewed in axial, or transverse, planes. This plane can best be understood if the body is thought of as a loaf of bread. Each transverse image, or slice, is obtained individually, without imaging of the other slices. Axial images of the human body are viewed as if the examiner were standing at the patient's feet, looking up through the body toward the head.

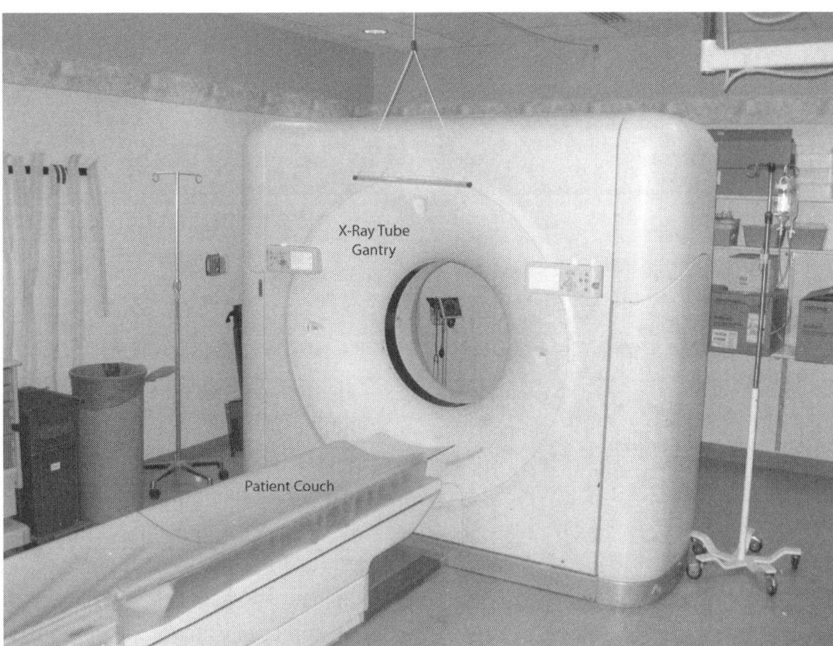

Figure 3-8. Standard computed tomography (CT) equipment. (Image courtesy of Cory Duncan.)

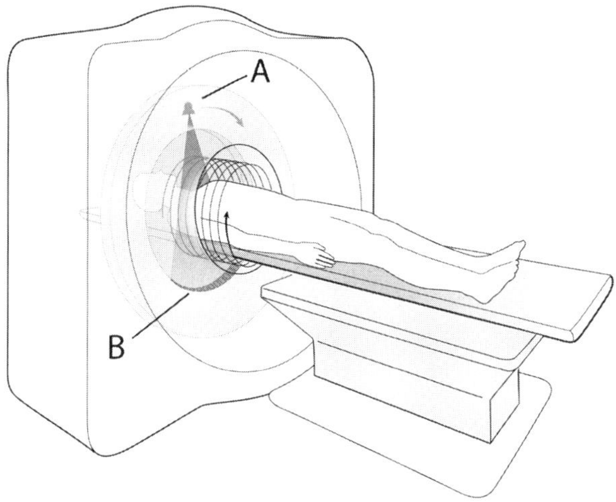

Figure 3-9. Typical computed tomography (CT) imaging process. The image shows the rotating path of the fan-shaped x-ray beam (A) and detector row (B), as well as patient movement through the gantry. (Image courtesy of Cory Duncan.)

Advances in computer science and programming have changed the way we view images reconstructed by CT software. Knowing the actual attenuation at each point in the body makes it possible for images to be reconstructed in multiple planes. Classically, images are viewed in the axial (transverse) plane. Today, it is common for reconstructed images to be provided in sagittal and coronal planes as well (Figure 3-10). These viewing planes are named after the suture lines in the skull where individual bones fuse to form the solid cranium.

The sagittal plane is named for the sagittal suture in the skull, which divides the skull into right and left halves. Sagittal images split the body into right and left pieces and are viewed as if the examiner were looking into the body from the side. The coronal plane is named for the coronal suture, which traverses the top of the skull from right to left. Coronal images divide the body into front and back (anterior and posterior) portions and are viewed as if one were looking into the body from the front.

As with plain film radiography, x-ray beams passing through the body during a CT scan are absorbed, attenuated, and scattered relative to tissue density. Instead of exposing radiographic film, the x-rays produced by CT scanners strike a detector and are converted to an

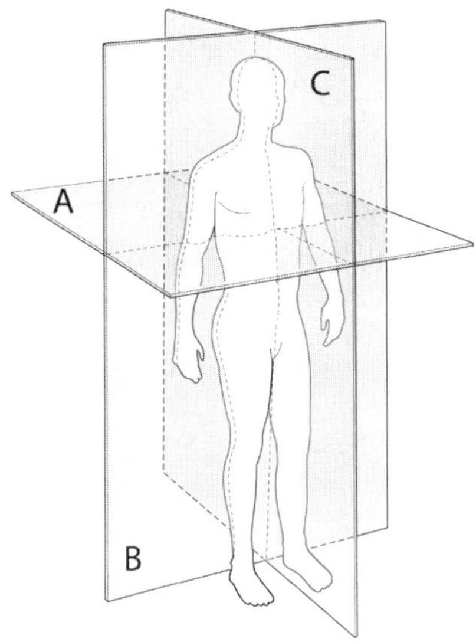

Figure 3-10. Transverse (A), coronal (B), and sagittal (C) imaging planes used in computed tomography (CT). (Image courtesy of Cory Duncan.)

electric current that is digitized and referred to in CT units or Hounsfield units (HU). This energy is converted into shades of black, gray, and white depending on tissue density. X-rays that pass freely to the detector through air will be converted to black images. Conversely, a dense structure like bone will absorb most of the x-ray beam, and the paucity of energy registered by the detector will result in a white image. Soft tissues will appear gray depending on the amount of absorption, attenuation, and scatter that is encountered (Figure 3-11A).

An advantage of the computerized image processing used in CT scanning is the ability to view the obtained images in different "window levels." Viewing images in different window levels is a departure from the traditional way of viewing images in shades of black, gray, and white. In CT scanning, the actual attenuation of each pixel (in Hounsfield units) on the screen is known relative to the others on the basis of tissue density. Computer processing can optimize the image for preferential viewing of certain structures. "Lung windows" are commonly used in chest imaging to better evaluate the soft tissues in the lungs. "Bone windows" are used throughout the body to evaluate the integrity of osseous structures. "Blood windows" highlight the acute accumulation of blood in the skull after trauma or hemorrhage (Figures 3-11A and 3-11B).

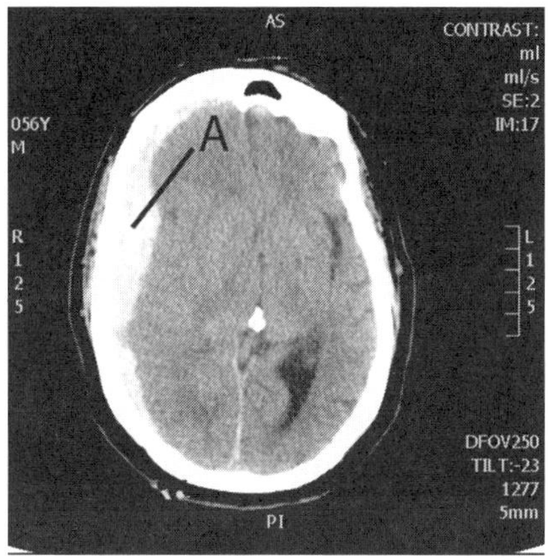

Figure 3-11A. CT image of head in "soft-tissue" window level showing large subdural hematoma (A) compressing the patient's right cerebral hemisphere. (Image courtesy of Cory Duncan.)

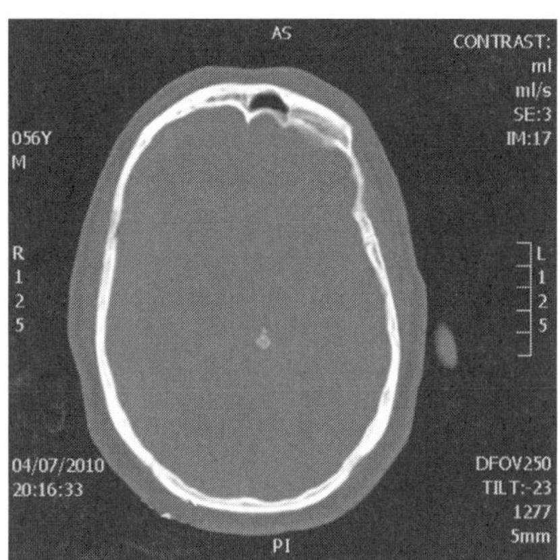

Figure 3-11B. Head CT obtained using the "bone" window. This image is the same anatomic slice as the image in Figure 3-11A. Computer processing has optimized the image for evaluation of osseous structures. (Image courtesy of Cory Duncan.)

Intravenous (IV) contrast agents are radiopaque and increase the density of blood vessels. Frequently they are given to patients during a CT scan to optimize visualization of large blood vessels and highly vascular areas of the body. IV contrast is used to evaluate the aorta and other large blood vessels for trauma, occlusion, and other disease. Areas where a pathologic process (e.g., infection, neoplasm) is receiving increased blood flow will be enhanced and better visualized with the use of IV contrast. Orally administered contrast agents can also be given during CT scanning of the abdomen and pelvis to delineate the contrast-filled bowel from other soft-tissue structures in the abdomen.

Recent advances in imaging technology have led to the development of CT scanners that obtain images quickly and with greater tissue differentiation. *High-resolution CT* is used to obtain images of the body in intervals as small as 1.0 mm. This is commonly used for the evaluation of parenchymal lung disease. *Helical CT,* also known as *spiral CT,* is frequently used and involves the patient being continuously transported through the gantry while the x-ray tube constantly rotates around the patient. Visually, it appears as if the x-ray tube is following a helical orbit around the patient, like a corkscrew. Helical CT scanning results in better image quality than conventional CT imaging because of higher resolution and sharper color contrast.

Helical CT scanners can be outfitted with multiple rows of x-ray tube/detector assemblies and allow extremely fast image capture rates as the patient constantly moves through the gantry. The newest *multislice CT* scanners have as many as 256 detector rings in one unit, allowing large areas of the body to be imaged in one rotation of the gantry. Multislice CT scanning can efficiently capture images that have limited motion artifact and high spatial resolution. Because of the high volume of images obtained in one rotation, multislice CT scanning can generate both static and cine images. This has been extremely useful in CT angiography, where enhanced visualization of large blood vessels and arterial trees is possible following IV contrast administration. CT angiography is commonly used in place of traditional angiography to evaluate the aorta and major branches, carotid arteries in the neck, cerebral vasculature, and arterial structures in the extremities following trauma.

Radiation Exposure

The use of x-rays as a diagnostic tool in medical practice today is well established. Radiography, fluoroscopy, and CT are modalities that utilize x-rays in screening for illness, diagnosing disease, and monitoring health. Unfortunately, the benefits these imaging procedures provide do not come without a risk to patient health. X-rays are a form of ionizing radiation, and even at low doses they may damage or destroy cells in ways that lead to solid cancers and leukemia. A common way of monitoring nonhomogeneous exposures to ionizing radiation is by the *effective dose.* Effective dose is measured in sieverts (Sv), an estimate of the overall harm caused by radiation exposure.

Exposure to the ionizing radiation used in radiologic procedures is not limited to the patients. Individuals at risk for repeated exposure, such as workers in the health care and nuclear industries, are continuously monitored. Typically, they are limited to effective doses of 20 mSv every year, not to exceed 100 mSv in 5 years or 50 mSv in any single year.[6] Unfortunately, patients undergoing radiologic procedures are not monitored.

In 2007, it was estimated that over 60 million CT scans were obtained in the United States. This is roughly a 20-fold increase from the estimated 3 million scans obtained in 1980.[7] Radiologic procedures have become the main source of effective dose radiation to which individuals in the United States are exposed. CT is rapid, simple, and accurate in the screening of asymptomatic patients and diagnosis of symptomatic patients. As a result, the use of CT, and therefore the exposure to radiation, will continue to rise. Currently, CT is being evaluated as a noninvasive means of screening the heart, lungs, colon, and whole body for disease.

Recently, two important longitudinal studies have evaluated the effects of radiation exposure on atomic bomb survivors in Japan and radiation workers in the nuclear industry. Atomic bomb survivors who received low doses of radiation, from 5 to 150 mSv (average 40 mSv), were at a significant overall risk for cancer.[8] This would be the equivalent of two or three CT scans in an adult (Table 3-1).

As medical and radiologic technology advances, it becomes easier for clinicians to use rapid, noninvasive imaging procedures in the screening, diagnosis, and treatment of disease. Recent literature has proved that there is a link between carcinomas and cumulative radiation exposure

Table 3-1. Typical Effective Radiation Doses from Various Radiologic Studies[7,8]

Study Type	Average Effective Dose (mSv)
Dental radiograph	0.005
Chest radiograph	0.02
Mammography	0.4
CT of head	2
CT of chest	7
CT angiography of chest	15
CT of abdomen and pelvis	14
Cardiac catheterization	15
Myocardial perfusion imaging	15.6
Neonatal abdominal CT	20

over a lifetime. The benefits of radiologic procedures that expose individuals to harmful ionizing radiation must be weighed against the long-term risk.

References

1. Hendee WR, Ritenour ER. *Medical Imaging Physics.* 4th ed. New York: Wiley-Liss; 2002.
2. DiSantis DJ. Early American radiology: the pioneer years. *AJR Am J Roentgenol.* 1986;147:850–3.
3. Goodman PC. The new light: discovery and introduction of the X-ray. *AJR Am J Roentgenol.* 1995;165:1041–5.
4. Suetens P. *Fundamentals of Medical Imaging.* Cambridge, UK; New York: Cambridge University Press; 2002.
5. Erkonen WE, Smith WL. *Radiology 101: The Basics and Fundamentals of Imaging.* 3rd ed. Philadelphia: Wolters Kluwer/Lippincott Williams & Wilkins Health; 2009.
6. Fazel R, Krumholz HM, Wang Y, et al. Exposure to low-dose ionizing radiation from medical imaging procedures. *N Engl J Med.* 2009;361:849–57.
7. Hall EJ, Brenner DJ. Cancer risks from diagnostic radiology. *Br J Radiol.* 2008; 81:362–78.
8. Brenner DJ, Hall EJ. Computed tomography—an increasing source of radiation exposure. *N Engl J Med.* 2007;357:2277–84.

CHAPTER 4

Adjunct Agents Used in X-Ray Imaging

Contrast Media

Vivian S. Loveless

History

Wilhelm Conrad Roentgen reported his discovery of x-rays in late 1895. It was noted immediately that these first x-ray images were limited—with the exception of those images in which there was defined contrast between soft tissues and bone or gastrointestinal (GI) gas. By the following March, visualization of a dead guinea pig's stomach was accomplished through intragastric instillation of a radiopaque (radiocontrast) agent, lead acetate. Concurrently, imaging of a human patient's esophagus and stomach was accomplished through oral administration of bismuth subnitrate, which became the standard radiocontrast pharmaceutical for evaluating the alimentary tract at that time.[1]

Although bismuth subnitrate provided outstanding radiocontrast, numerous problems were associated with its use. The problems included the instability of aqueous preparations of bismuth compounds as well as undesired effects on patients: neurologic abnormalities, GI irritation, and methemoglobinemia. In addition, during World War I, supply chain issues occurred when the supply of bismuth from Europe was halted. Beginning in 1914, the choice of radiopaque contrast agent for gastric imaging shifted from bismuth to barium sulfate,[1] which continues to have widespread use today.

In addition to its use for GI imaging, before 1906 bismuth subnitrate was administered via retrograde instillation into the lower urinary tract for the purpose of demonstrating the urinary system; however, administration by this route also was fraught with problems. Successful imaging was accomplished in 1906 with instillation of a silver compound into the urinary tract, but it was discovered that silver compounds caused renal toxicity with effects ranging from renal necrosis to death. Important advances in retrograde urography occurred with the use of sodium and potassium iodides in 1917 and with a 20% solution of sodium bromide around 1918. The first organic iodide radiopaque drug was Lipiodol, which was used successfully in 1922 to obtain radiographic images. This agent also had toxicity and adverse reaction issues that limited its use.[1] Since these early attempts to use radiopaque agents as a supplement to x-ray imaging, many advances have been made in the development of radiopaque agents and in the methods of administration, enabling the desired information to be obtained with reduced toxicity and fewer adverse reactions.

Contrast Role in Imaging

Contrast agents are used in x-ray procedures, magnetic resonance (MR) imaging, and ultrasound imaging procedures. Today, radiopaque contrast media (ROCM), such as barium and iodine, are used to facilitate x-ray imaging of internal organs. The atomic number (Z) and mass density of both barium ($Z = 56$) and iodine ($Z = 53$) are much higher than those of soft tissue ($Z = 7.4$). Since these elements have a high Z, they are designated as positive contrast agents,[2] meaning they attenuate x-rays to a greater degree than do soft tissues of the body. Iodinated agents are soluble in water, whereas barium agents are not.[3] For example, when an artery is filled with an iodinated compound it can be easily observed on a radiograph. Similarly, the colon can be visualized when it is filled with barium.

Negative contrast agents attenuate x-rays to a lesser extent than do soft tissues of the body.[3] In some x-ray examinations of the colon, air can be used as a negative contrast agent while barium serves as the positive contrast agent.[2] Currently, no negative contrast agents are commercially available as approved pharmaceuticals,[3] although there are several sources for medical-grade gases that are approved for human use. When both positive and negative contrast are used together, the examination is known as a double-contrast examination.[2]

Contrast agents have the advantage of augmenting the differences between body tissues shown on images by modifying tissue response to x-ray energy. The disadvantage to the use of contrast agents lies in the adverse effects elicited by these compounds.[3]

Intravascular Radiographic Contrast Media

Iodine-based contrast agents can be used during conventional radiography, computed tomography (CT), and angiography. Because the blood vessels and the blood flowing through the vessels possess densities comparable to those of the surrounding soft tissues, it is necessary to inject contrast media in order to perform angiographic procedures.[4] Intravascular radiographic (radiopaque) contrast agents can be administered either intravenously or intra-arterially for the purpose of providing increased density to vascular structures to augment the anatomic image.[5] The basic structure of these contrast agents is a benzene ring with three iodine atoms attached. Some ROCM are considered to be monomers, containing a single benzene ring, whereas others are dimers consisting of two benzene rings.[3]

Intravascular ROCM can be divided into four groups: high-osmolality ionic, low-osmolality ionic, low-osmolality nonionic, and iso-osmolality nonionic contrast agents. Iso-osmolality agents have a lower osmolality than low-osmolality agents.[6] The method by which an agent becomes water soluble is related to whether the agent is ionic or nonionic. In the body, water is unevenly polarized, with negative poles around the oxygen atoms and positive poles around the hydrogen atoms. Since ionic contrast media separate into cations and anions after intravascular administration, they attract negative and positive poles of water molecules and so are soluble in water. In contrast, nonionic ROCM do not separate into positive and negative ions after intravascular administration; rather, they are made water soluble by their polar OH groups. There is a force of attraction between the electrical poles in the OH groups of nonionic ROCM and the electrical poles of the water molecules.[3] The contrast ratio determines the osmolality of ROCM; this ratio equals the number of iodine atoms divided by the number of particles in solution.[3] The number of particles in solution is determined by whether the agent is ionic or nonionic. Ionic agents would have two particles in solution (positive and negative ions), while nonionic ROCM would only have one osmotically active particle.[5] As stated earlier, ROCM having two benzene rings are considered dimers, while ROCM with only one benzene ring are considered monomers. Since each benzene ring has three iodine atoms attached, it is easy to understand the concept of contrast agent ratio.[3] For example, the ratio of an ionic contrast agent that is a monomer is calculated as follows:

$$1.5 = \frac{\text{3 iodine atoms}}{\text{2 particles}}$$

The ratio calculation for a nonionic dimer is

$$6 = \frac{\text{6 iodine atoms}}{\text{1 particle}}$$

The ratio calculation for an ionic dimer is

$$3 = \frac{\text{6 iodine atoms}}{\text{2 particles}}$$

The ratio calculation for a nonionic monomer is

$$3 = \frac{\text{3 iodine atoms}}{\text{1 particle}}$$

The ROCM with lower ratios, like the ionic monomer agents, tend to have higher osmolality (more particles per iodine atom). The iso-osmolality agents are the nonionic dimers, whereas low-osmolality ROCM include ionic dimers and nonionic monomers.[3] Table 4-1 provides examples of the four categories of ROCM.

Dosage and Administration

Iodinated contrast agents are used in a wide variety of diagnostic imaging procedures looking at most of the major organ systems in the body. Most of the contrast agents are described by the name of the iodine-containing molecule (e.g., diatrizoate, iothalamate), but they are also described by the number of milligrams of bound iodine per milliliter

Table 4-1. Categories of Radiopaque Contrast Media[3,5]

Class	General Structure	Examples (Iodine-Containing Component)
High-osmolality ionic	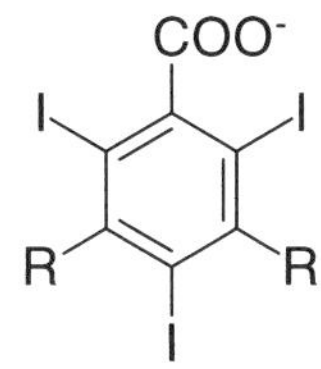	Diatrizoate Iothalamate
Low-osmolality ionic	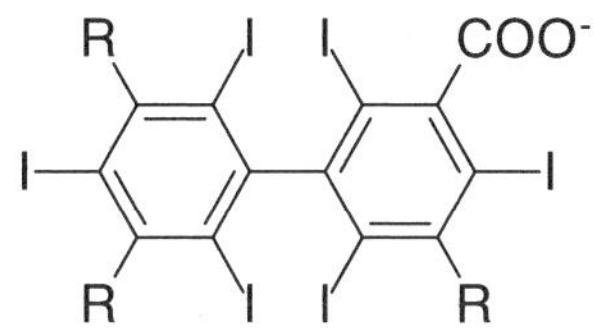	Ioxaglate meglumine
Low-osmolality nonionic	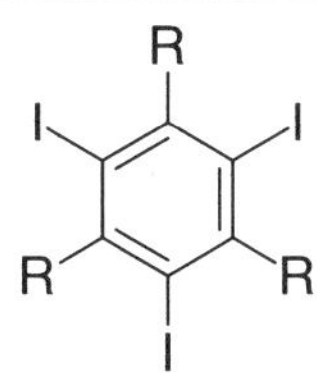	Iodipamide Iohexol Iopamidol Iopromide Ioversol
Iso-osmolality nonionic	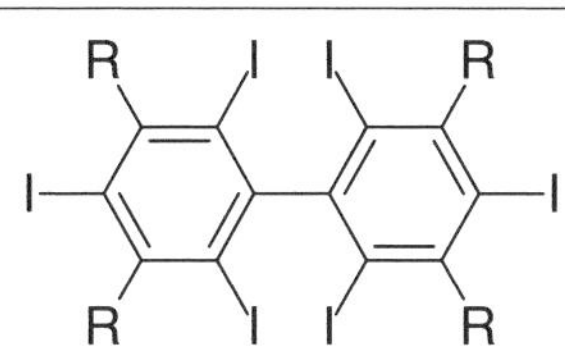	Iodixanol

of solution. This information is commonly found in the package insert. Some of the trade names for iodinated contrast media suggest the body part for which that agent is approved—for example, Cystografin (diatrizoate meglumine [Bracco]) and Renografin (diatrizoate meglumine–diatrizoate sodium [Bracco]) are indicated for studies of the urinary bladder and the renal system—whereas many of the agents have multiple indications. When administered by the intravenous route, all contrast media are distributed in the extracellular space and will predominantly be excreted renally,[5] primarily by glomerular filtration.[7] There are no significant differences in pharmacokinetics, pharmacodynamics, or clinical efficacy among agents in the low-osmolar iodinated contrast media category, so most institutions will have a small selection of contrast agents available on their formulary.[7] Contrast agents for use in adults are usually dosed by volume, depending on the study and the area of the body being imaged. Pediatric doses are determined on a volume per kilogram of body weight basis.[8–12]

Adverse Reactions

The adverse effects caused by iodinated ROCM result to some degree from their osmolality and the tissue or serum concentration of iodine, calcium-chelating ability, anticoagulant properties, and immune system-stimulating capability.[13] There appear to be no significant differences between the adverse effect profiles of agents within a particular class.[7] Many patients receiving intravascular ROCM have subjective sensations such as altered taste, flushing, and warmth, which last only a few minutes and are clinically insignificant. The administration of intravascular ROCM can also lead to the development of acute idiosyncratic reactions, which can be classified as mild, moderate, or severe. Mild reactions do not routinely require treatment; examples are itching, urticaria, nausea, and mild vomiting. Vasovagal reactions, facial or laryngeal edema, bronchospasm, marked urticaria, and more severe vomiting are examples of moderate reactions. Examples of severe reactions include cardiac arrest, convulsions, respiratory arrest, pulmonary edema, and hypotension.[14] Almost all acute, serious reactions have their onset within the first 20 minutes after administration of the ROCM.[7,14] An estimated 1 out of 20,000 to 40,000 patients administered ROCM dies as a result of serious adverse effects.[13] However, most adverse reactions are mild and no therapy or medication is needed beyond continued observation and reassurance of the patient.[15]

For most patients experiencing vasodilation and flushing after intravascular ROCM administration, the agents' osmolality is thought to be the cause. ROCM administration causes an increase in osmotic pressure intravascularly, which causes movement of tissue water into the vascular lumen for the purpose of dilution.[13] Soon after administration, the cardiovascular system dilutes the hyperosmolar contrast agent, resulting in an intravascular hypo-osmolar state in relation to the extravascular space. As a result of dehydration, the extravascular space is now hyperosmolar; thus, there is another fluid shift, this time from the intravascular lumen to the tissue space. These shifts between the extravascular and intravascular spaces continue until osmolar equilibrium is attained. The renal adverse reactions caused by these contrast agents may be partially due to these osmotic fluid shifts.[13]

Vasovagal reactions can occur when a hyperosmolar contrast agent is introduced into the carotid arteries, causing changes in the intra-arterial osmotic pressure. When the change is great enough to stimulate chemoreceptors and baroreceptors, the autonomic nervous system causes bradycardia, resulting in a decrease in aortic pressure.[13]

In patients with chronic congestive heart failure, acute heart failure can be induced by intravascular osmotic fluid shifts. To counteract this, diuretics (e.g., furosemide) can be used to cause fluid excretion, and cardiac stimulators (e.g., dobutamine) can be administered to strengthen the force of cardiac contraction.[13]

A small percentage of patients experience adverse cardiac rhythms after receiving intravascular ROCM. One causative factor may be chelation of calcium ions in the cardiovascular system. High-osmolality ROCM can produce anticoagulant effects; however, it is thought that this does not occur with low-osmolality agents.[13]

Acute idiosyncratic systemic reactions to contrast media are those characterized as unpredictable, occurring within 1 hour after administration, and unrelated to the quantity of administered contrast medium. These reactions have been described as "allergy-like" or anaphylactoid, but the causative mechanism remains unclear. However, data indicate that some severe acute reactions to iodinated contrast media are true allergic hypersensitivity reactions. Immediate significant increases in plasma histamine and tryptase have occurred in patients having severe acute reactions, and the increases were proportionate to the reaction severity. The timing and level of the increases were comparable to those seen in known allergic hypersensitivity reactions, suggesting that instantaneous degranulation of mast cells was taking place. The most significant factor predisposing a patient to an acute idiosyncratic reaction is a previous reaction to ROCM. The reported risk of a reaction to an ionic ROCM in a patient who previously reacted to this type of ROCM ranges from 16% to 35%. However, when a patient who previously had a reaction to an ionic ROCM is administered a nonionic ROCM, there is only about a 5% risk of a repeat reaction.[14] Table 4-2 lists some of the drugs that can be used in the treatment of anaphylactic reactions.

Table 4-2. Drugs Used to Treat Anaphylactic Reactions[15]

Epinephrine
Aminophylline
Diphenhydramine
Corticosteroids
Physiologic IV fluids

It has been postulated that direct chemotoxicity could produce immediate nonallergic effects of ROCM.[14] Mediating factors for this effect include dose or concentration, site of and rate of injection, osmolality, formulation, viscosity, and molecular toxicity.[15]

Another type of reaction that can occur is an anaphylactoid reaction. Even though it mimics clinically an anaphylactic reaction, no previous exposure to iodinated contrast media is needed to sensitize the mast cells. The mast cells can release their chemicals on the very first exposure to an iodinated contrast agent. It should be kept in mind that a reaction of this type can be as lethal as an anaphylactic reaction.[13]

About 10% of all cases of acute renal failure (ARF) are the result of ROCM administration.[9] Contrast-induced nephropathy (CIN) occurs when there is an increase in serum creatinine by 25% or by more than 0.5 mg/dL within 72 hours of contrast administration.[16] Patients with preexisting renal dysfunction (serum creatinine in excess of 1.5 mg/dL), especially when renal impairment is due to diabetic nephropathy, are at the greatest risk for developing ARF as a result of contrast media administration. Without renal impairment, diabetes mellitus is not a risk factor for ROCM-induced ARF. The level of renal impairment existing prior to ROCM administration dictates the severity of the nephropathy caused by ROCM. Since dehydration and congestive heart failure are associated with decreased renal perfusion, they are considered risk factors for ischemic insult to the kidneys by ROCM administration.[17] If a patient is dehydrated prior to ROCM administration, it is imperative that the patient be hydrated after the study to avoid significant ARF. The frequency of ARF reported after angiography is 2%, compared with 2% to 25% in patients undergoing intravenous pyelography. Of diabetic patients with renal nephropathy, 50% to 100% can experience ARF after administration of ROCM.[13] Patients with normal renal function are at fairly low risk for developing CIN, [17] and the risk increases with worsening renal function. For patients who are at risk for developing CIN, the American College of Radiology and Consensus Panel for CIN suggest several precautions that should be considered. Ideally, the patients should be adequately hydrated, with supplemental hydration in the 12 hours before administration and continuing for 6 hours after ROCM administration. Low-osmolar or iso-osmolar contrast agents should be used if at all possible. Medications that may adversely affect renal function should be withheld prior to and immediately after the imaging study.[18] The nephrotoxic effects of ROCM can be enhanced in patients receiving nephrotoxic drugs, such as aminoglycosides and non-steroidal anti-inflammatory drugs (NSAIDs). High-osmolality ROCM are more nephrotoxic than low-osmolality and iso-osmolality agents.[17]

ARF caused by administration of ROCM can present either as an oliguric (urine output not greater than 400 mL/day) or a nonoliguric reaction. In general, patients are more likely to have nonoliguric ARF that is reversible and of limited duration. The serum creatinine level becomes elevated in the first 24 hours after administration, peaks in 2 to 4 days, and returns to normal by 7 to 10 days. Oliguric ARF, however, may not be reversible.[13] Drugs used to prevent renal impairment in patients receiving ROCM are listed in Table 4-3.

Thyroid storm is a rare adverse effect of ROCM, but it is potentially fatal. The patients most likely to experience this event are those with decompensated thyrotoxicosis. The iodine in the ROCM can result in the release of thyroid hormones in amounts exceeding these patients' tolerance level. Even thyroid hormone levels considered to be normal can exceed the tolerance level for this group of patients.[13]

Katayama et al.[19] reported a higher frequency of adverse drug reactions in patients receiving ionic contrast media than in those receiving nonionic media, as well as a decreased rate of severe adverse events with nonionic ROCM. Ho et al.[6] compared the rate of adverse events when iodixanol (a nonionic, iso-osmolar contrast agent) was used in CT studies with the rate for iohexol (a nonionic, low-osmolality agent) in CT studies. The iodixanol group had 15,142 patients and the iohexol group had 22,044 patients. Fewer than 1% of patients in either group experienced adverse reactions; however, there was a significantly greater rate of both immediate and delayed adverse reactions with iodixanol than with iohexol.

Contraindications

Contrast agents are contraindicated in patients who have experienced severe reactions to previous administration of these agents and in patients with severe renal dysfunction. Ionic contrast agents are contraindicated for

Table 4-3. Drugs Used to Prevent Renal Impairment in Patients Receiving ROCM[13,17]

Drug	Dosage and Frequency	Indication
0.9% or 0.45% sodium chloride injection	1–1.5 mL/kg IV 12 hours before the exam and continuing for at least 24 hours after the exam[a]	Hydration to prevent dehydration
Fenoldopam	Titrated beginning at 0.03 μg/kg/min IV and increasing to 0.1 μg/kg/min by 1–2 hours before angiography and continuing for a minimum of 6 hours[b]	Vasodilatory effects
Acetylcysteine	600 mg orally beginning 12 hours before procedure and continued every 12 hours for 2 days[c]	Antioxidant; possibly a vasodilator
Sodium bicarbonate	3 mL/kg/hr IV of solution (154 mEq sodium bicarbonate in 1000 mL 5% dextrose injection) 1 hour before administration of ROCM, then decreasing to 1 mL/kg/hr during exam and continuing for 6 hours after procedure at 1 mL/kg/hr	Alter pH of urine to prevent formation of toxic free ionic radicals

[a] Should be used only if patient's cardiac health permits.
[b] Titration conducted at 15–20 minute intervals; administration stopped if systolic blood pressure drops to less than 99 mm Hg.
[c] To administer, add to soda or juice to mask unpalatable taste and smell.

intrathecal administration, as they are unsuitable for direct contact with neural tissue. Following intravenous administration, the blood–brain barrier appears to protect neural tissue from these effects, but intrathecal administration can result in severe muscle spasms, seizures, cerebral edema, and cerebral hemorrhage, progressing to death. Nonionic agents are significantly less neurotoxic and are used for intrathecal administration.[20]

Medication Therapy Management (MTM) Concerns

Patients should be screened prior to administration of contrast media for certain risk factors that may indicate a higher likelihood of adverse effects. Patients with a history of adverse reactions to contrast media or serious allergic reactions to agents other than contrast media, a history of asthma, known cardiac issues, or renal insufficiency should be thoroughly evaluated before administration of these agents. Patients' medication profiles should be evaluated thoroughly prior to administration to screen for agents that potentially could contribute to adverse effects or that should be avoided when contrast agents are administered.[7]

Even though ROCM are not considered highly active pharmacologically,[21] they may alter the pharmacologic action of traditional pharmaceuticals.[4,21] ROCM can interact with both traditional drugs and radiopharmaceuticals.[21]

When a patient's renal function is altered by ROCM, the pharmacokinetics of other pharmaceuticals, especially those eliminated renally, can be altered. When a contrast agent induces a decrease in renal function, this can cause retention of drugs excreted entirely via the kidneys. Metformin can be retained when contrast media cause an impairment of renal function, which can lead to lactic acidosis, a serious complication.[21] Metformin should be discontinued 48 hours prior to the study[22] and withheld for a minimum of 48 hours after completion of the imaging study;[23] ideally, renal function should be assessed before restarting this medication.[22]

When a patient taking methotrexate undergoes an exam with ROCM, there can be an additive nephrotoxic effect. Since methotrexate is eliminated renally, nephrotoxicity can cause retention of methotrexate, resulting in toxicity. ROCM are contraindicated in patients receiving a high dosage of methotrexate and having a methotrexate serum concentration of >0.1 μmol/L. When the serum concentration of methotrexate is less than 0.1 μmol/L, ROCM should be used cautiously and only the smallest dose of an iso-osmolality or low-osmolality contrast medium should be administered. It is recommended that intravenous hydration with normal saline (0.9% sodium chloride injection) be used for a minimum of 6 hours before and 6 hours after ROCM administration.[21]

NSAIDs can compound the adverse renal effects of ROCM by enhancing the contrast agents' renal vasoconstrictor effect, thus aiding in the development of ROCM-induced nephrotoxicity.[21] This occurs because of NSAIDs' interference with the synthesis of vasodilatory prostaglandins in the renal system. Other drugs enhancing the nephrotoxic effects of ROCM include aminoglycosides, amphotericin, rifampin, lithium carbonate, and antineoplastics. Diuretics such as furosemide, thiazides, triamterene, amiloride, ethacrynic acid, and spironolactone can enhance the hypotensive and diuretic effects of ROCM. The outcome can be dehydration leading to increased risk of ROCM-induced nephropathy and electrolyte imbalance. Also, heightened and prolonged hypotensive effects can occur. Hypokalemia caused by the diuretics can, in conjunction with ROCM, produce additive prolongation of the QT interval, which can cause ventricular tachycardia.[4]

Drugs that augment allergy-like reactions to ROCM include β-adrenergic-receptor blocking agents, interleukins, and interferon. In patients taking hydralazine, ROCM should be avoided because cutaneous vasculitis can occur several hours after intravascular injection of nonionic contrast media.[21] Beta-blockers can interact with ROCM to heighten and lengthen hypotensive effects.[4] In one study, 1.8% of patients who had received interleukin-2 and undergone a CT exam with ROCM experienced urticarial reactions within 1 hour of ROCM administration.[21] In this same study, 12% of patients experienced delayed reactions (e.g., flulike symptoms, pruritus, erythema, rash, fever, flushing); the mean time of onset of the reactions was 4.5 hours and the mean duration of symptoms was 16.4 hours. The time since interleukin-2 therapy ranged from 24 days to 2.4 years. There is an increased risk of ROCM-induced reactions for as long as 2 years after cessation of interleukin-2 therapy. A relative contraindication to additional ROCM administration exists when a patient on interleukin-2 has had a previous reaction to ROCM. It should also be noted that ROCM may precipitate interleukin-2 toxicity.

Since iodinated ROCM can prolong clotting time, the effects of anticoagulants and antiplatelet drugs can be exaggerated. Calcium-channel blocking agents in combination with ionic high-osmolar ROCM can result in hypotension. Ionic high-osmolar iodinated contrast media can also cause peripheral vasodilatation and produce a negative inotropic effect on the heart. However, this is not a significant problem with the modern nonionic, low-osmolar iodinated ROCM, since these have a minimal negative inotropic myocardial effect and are less vasoactive.[21]

The free iodide in the ROCM interferes with both diagnostic scintigraphy and radioiodine therapy by decreasing the uptake of radioiodine radiopharmaceuticals.[21] Scintigraphy should be delayed between 1 and 6 weeks after administration of water-soluble ROCM, depending on the indication for scintigraphy and the thyroid status of the patient.[21,24]

It is recommended that erythrocyte labeling with technetium ^{99m}Tc not be conducted within 24 hours of administration of ROCM.[21]

It is not advisable for ROCM to be mixed with traditional drugs prior to intravascular administration, because the mixture may alter the stability of the drugs.[21] Traditional drugs can interact with ROCM to form chemical incompatibilities that can result in insoluble precipitates with the potential to occlude intravenous catheters and possibly cause an embolism that could block small vessels. Depending on which vessel is blocked, the consequences could range from mild to fatal.[13] Thus, using the same venous access for ROCM and other pharmaceuticals is not recommended.[21] If the same access must be used, then the site must be adequately flushed with 0.9% sodium chloride injection between injections.[13,21]

Enteral Contrast Agents

Radiologic studies of the GI tract are used for numerous indications: GI bleeding, abdominal pain, distinct alterations in bowel habits, and other digestive tract disorders.[25] Another use for enteral contrast agents is to assist in defining the cardiac shadow.[5] Enteral contrast agents are either barium suspensions or iodine solutions.

Barium Sulfate

Dosage and Administration

The dosage form for barium sulfate is a suspension of insoluble barium sulfate particles,[3] and this contrast medium can be given orally or rectally as an adjunct to the diagnosis of disorders of the GI tract.[5] Since pure barium sulfate suspension flocculates readily and yields inadequate mucosal coating, additives are used in the commercial preparations to improve the suspension's mucosal coating properties, avoid flocculation, and enhance palatability for oral use. Some of the additives used are carboxymethyl cellulose, agar-agar, pectin, and sorbitol; however, the literature describes more than 90 different additives.[26] Immediately after oral administration, radiodensity occurs in the esophagus and stomach; however, radiodensity of the duodenum may require 15 to 90 minutes after administration. After rectal administration, radiodensity is observed in the rectum and colon immediately.[5]

Barium sulfate preparations are commercially available in a variety of formulations such as suspensions, powders for suspension, tablets, and suspension paste.[27] Final formulations of these products vary significantly in regard to viscosity, density, and regional GI stability. These physical properties are related to the concentration and nature of the various additives as well as to the concentration, uniformity, and size of the barium sulfate particles. The density and stability of the barium contrast medium is dependent on the relative size, shape, and uniformity of the product's barium sulfate particles.[25]

Manufacturers list concentrations of barium sulfate suspensions as either percent weight in volume (% w/v) or percent by weight (% w/w). Concentrations vary among the various formulations. The number of grams of barium sulfate in 100 mL of final suspension is designated as percent weight in volume, whereas the number of grams of barium sulfate in 100 grams of the final suspension is listed as percent by weight. In addition, percent by weight is used in reference to barium sulfate powders; the percentage designates the total powder weight resulting from pure barium sulfate versus the weight of the solid additives.[25]

A barium sulfate medium's density can be estimated by dividing the percent weight in weight concentration into the percent weight in volume concentration. The preparation's density can also be thought of in terms of the ratio of measured volume occupied by barium sulfate particles to the proportion occupied by "voids" (e.g., additives, water, air, or combinations of these). Preparations with a low density have a high percentage of voids. The size and uniformity of the barium sulfate particles in suspension influence the density and the proportion of voids. Preparations with the largest proportion of voids have the least number of contact points, and this occurs with uniform size particles. Preparations containing large, nonuniform particles are the densest barium sulfate media. The density of the barium sulfate contrast medium and the total volume of medium directly in the x-ray beam path determine the degree of radiopacification resulting from the administration of this medium. To facilitate sufficient opacification in a double-contrast study when the mucosal surface is only thinly coated, a high-density barium sulfate medium is necessary. A low-density barium sulfate medium is required for the increased thickness of a full-column, single-contrast study. In a single-contrast study with a barium sulfate preparation of excessive density, there is the potential to obscure some lesions because sufficient penetration by the x-rays could be hindered.[25]

The measure of the barium sulfate medium's resistance to flow is known as its viscosity. The viscosity plays a significant role in determining how the medium is used and its stability. The viscosity of the medium is directly related to barium sulfate's concentration in suspension but inversely proportional to the temperature of the agent. An increase in viscosity occurs if there are very small particles present, since they have an increased surface area for adsorption of water and air. Some of the factors that influence the settling rate of a barium sulfate suspension are the medium's viscosity, particle size, and barium sulfate concentration. A barium sulfate formulation with an increased viscosity has a lower rate of particle settling. The stability of both single-contrast and double-contrast barium formulations is highly dependent on viscosity.[25]

A problem that can occur if the preparation's viscosity is too low is deposition and retention of only a very thin coating on the surface of the mucosa, with the result being insufficient opacification and an inclination to form a "weak spot" and rapid breakdown of the film. In contrast, when the medium is excessively viscous, it will not readily flow and there may be incomplete or nonuniform coating of the mucosa. Also, lesions on the mucosal surface could be obscured if too thick a coating is deposited.[25]

When a single-contrast study is conducted, it is necessary to have full-column opacification and distention of the segmental lumen being evaluated. This is accomplished by giving a large volume of a low-density barium sulfate formulation. Conversely, in a double-contrast study, a relatively small volume of a high-density, low-viscosity barium sulfate preparation is administered to achieve coating of the mucosal surface under investigation. In a double-contrast study, opacification of specific mucosal surface and demarcation of fine surface detail result from distention of the lumen through administration of a gas (a negative-contrast agent).[25]

Usually, the preferred ROCM for the GI tract is barium sulfate, since it gives a thorough demonstration of structures, particularly the mucosa, without causing widespread local adverse reactions. However, barium sulfate is not the preferred agent in a CT study of the GI tract, because it can be a source of significant artifact.[5]

After oral or rectal administration, there is negligible absorption of barium sulfate from the GI tract, resulting in excretion via feces in an unchanged form. The elimination rate is dependent on the administration route, status of the patient's peristaltic activity, and motility of the GI tract. Barium sulfate given orally is routinely eliminated within 24 hours in a normal patient. When given rectally, barium sulfate is excreted via evacuation of the enema,[25] which occurs at the completion of the imaging study.

Adverse Reactions

After either oral or rectal administration, colonic retention and delayed elimination of barium sulfate can occur if decreased intestinal motility is an issue.[25] Barium sulfate is usually safe; however, constipation and abdominal pain can follow oral or rectal administration. The primary risk is that barium may be retained in the colon for 6 weeks or more in patients with partial colonic obstruction or in elderly patients. After a barium enema enters the distal loop of a colostomy, there may be prolonged stasis of barium.[26] Formation of barium fecaliths capable of causing intestinal obstruction can result, because the colon's normal reabsorptive processes lead to dehydration of the barium sulfate remaining after evacuation.[25] Barium fecaliths are a rare complication and are generally observed in diverticula in the colon. They are frequently asymptomatic but may be related to bowel obstruction, bowel perforation, abdominal pain, or appendicitis. Surgical removal is sometimes necessary. Other adverse effects associated with barium preparations are listed in Table 4-4.[6]

Allergic reactions to barium-containing contrast agents are usually mild (pruritus, erythema, or urticaria) and respond to antihistamine administration. Severe allergic reactions require appropriate emergency measures.[28,29]

Table 4-4. Adverse Effects of Oral and Rectal Barium Contrast Media[4,6]

Aggravation of colonic toxic dilation
Leakage into the peritoneal cavity
Extravasation into the peritoneal cavity
Aspiration into the bronchial tree
Intravasation of suspension
Allergic reactions

Contraindications

Barium sulfate should not be used in patients with known or suspected obstructions in any area of the GI tract.[27–29] It should also be avoided in patients with known or suspected perforations in the bowel, to prevent escape of the insoluble barium suspension from the GI tract.[26–29] Patients with known hypersensitivity reactions to barium sulfate or any product component should not receive this contrast agent.[26,27] Barium sulfate suspensions contain a number of different additives, some of which have been reported to cause allergic responses in some patients.[26,30]

MTM Concerns

Because barium sulfate contrast media are unstable adsorption compounds that have the ability to bind to drugs, interaction of oral barium sulfate suspension with oral drugs having a narrow therapeutic margin is possible. The timing of administration of these drugs should be considered when the patient is scheduled for a barium contrast study. With normal biodistribution or retention of barium sulfate in the GI tract, there is potential for interference with other diagnostic procedures, such as other abdominal x-ray procedures or abdominal nuclear medicine studies.[25] Patients receiving oral barium should be monitored for vomiting or reflux that could lead to aspiration of the barium suspension into the respiratory tract and development of pneumonia, aspiration pneumonitis, or granulomas of the lung.[25–29,31]

Iodine Solutions

Dosage and Administration

The iodine solutions diatrizoate meglumine and diatrizoate sodium are indicated as contrast agents for evaluation of the GI tract. They can be administered either orally or rectally. These agents are indicated when there is concern that the administration of a barium sulfate suspension could cause harm, as in the case of a GI perforation. Because of these contrast agents' high osmolality, considerable osmotic activity occurs within the GI tract. When this occurs, the result is major iodine dilution and also copious diarrhea, dehydration, systemic hypovolemia, and imbalance of electrolytes. Barium sulfate is usually the preferred diagnostic agent for the GI tract, because iodine dilution produces less-definitive diagnostic exams and because of iodine's adverse effects.[5]

The oral dosage of an iodine-containing contrast agent may vary from 30 mL to 90 mL depending on the type of examination being performed and the size of the patient. For tomography, diluted preparations are indicated; for example, a common adult oral dosage is 240 mL of a diluted solution (25 mL of contrast medium diluted to 1 L with tap water). These agents can be administered orally to infants and children, although it is recommended that the products be diluted with water, carbonated beverages, milk, or mineral oil. Oral administration to elderly cachectic patients may also require dilution. For rectal administration of an iodinated preparation to an adult, the recommended dilution is 240 mL (88 grams of iodine) to 1 L with tap water.[32]

After rectal administration, there is prompt radiopacity in the rectum and colon; however, when an iodine agent is administered orally, 15 to 90 minutes may elapse before demonstration of radiopacity in the duodenum. After oral administration, radiodensity occurs promptly in the esophagus and stomach. ROCM for the GI tract do not cross the GI wall, so their biodistribution is limited to the GI lumen. Thus, these agents do not undergo metabolic activity, so they are eliminated with the feces.[5]

Adverse Reactions

Since the iodine-containing agents are sparingly absorbed from the GI tract, they elicit almost none of the physiologic effects associated with intravascular administration of these same contrast media. Health care professionals should be aware that even with very low systemic levels of iodinated contrast media, it is possible for pseudoallergic reactions to occur.[25] When a hypertonic contrast medium is administered enterally, the patient may develop hypovolemia and hypotension due to fluid loss through the intestine, which could result in a shocklike state in debilitated or young children and in elderly cachectic patients. Most adverse reactions are mild and transitory and include nausea, vomiting, and diarrhea; abdominal cramping; acute dyspnea; skin rashes; heartburn; dizziness; and headache. However, anaphylactic reactions have been reported, and it is theoretically possible for anaphylactoid reactions to occur after oral or rectal administration.[32]

Contraindications

Administration of iodine-containing contrast agents by the oral or rectal route is contraindicated for patients who have a known hypersensitivity to these agents or any components of these products.[32]

MTM Concerns

Because of their high iodine content, iodinated contrast agents should be administered with caution in patients with hyperthyroidism or euthyroid goiter. As with the barium agents, aspiration of iodine-containing contrast agents may lead to pulmonary complications including pulmonary edema, pneumonitis, or even death.[32,33] Patients with a history of a previous reaction to contrast agents and those with a known sensitivity to iodine or other clinical hypersensitivity conditions (e.g., asthma, food allergies) should be monitored carefully for signs of anaphylactoid or anaphylactic reactions following administration of these agents.[32]

Conclusion

Knowledge of the various types of ROCM will prepare pharmacists to be better able to provide pharmaceutical care to their patients. Pharmacists' awareness of the potential adverse effects and of drugs to prevent or treat these reactions will help ensure a positive patient outcome.

References

1. Barrs TJ. Overview of radiopaque drugs: 1895–1931. *Am J Health Syst Pharm.* 2006;63:2248–55.
2. Bushong SC. X-ray interaction with matter. In: Bushong SC, ed. *Radiologic Science for Technologists: Physics, Biology, and Protection.* 8th ed. St Louis: Elsevier Mosby; 2004:172–87.
3. Aspelin P, Bellin M-F, Jakobsen JA, et al. Classification and terminology. In: Thomsen HS, Webb JAW, eds. *Medical Radiology Diagnostic Imaging: Contrast Media Safety Issues and ESUR Guidelines.* 2nd ed. Berlin, Heidelberg: Springer-Verlag; 2009:3–9.
4. Swanson DP, Shetty PC, Kustan DJ, et al. Angiographic contrast media. In: Swanson DP, Chilton HM, Thrall JH, eds. *Pharmaceuticals in Medical Imaging.* New York: Macmillan; 1990:1–77.
5. Jensen SC, Peppers MP. Classification, chemistry, and pharmacology of contrast agents. In: Jensen SC, Peppers MP, eds. *Pharmacology and Drug Administration for Imaging Technologists.* 2nd ed. St Louis: Mosby Elsevier; 2006:64–80.
6. Ho AL, O'Malley ME, Tomlinson GA. Adverse events with universal use of iodixanol for CT: comparison with iohexol. *J Comput Assist Tomogr.* 2007;31:165–8.
7. American Society of Health-System Pharmacists. Quick guide to contrast media. Developed by ASHP Advantage. www.ashp.org/Import/PRACTICEANDPOLICY/PracticeResourceCenters/ContrastMedia/QuickGuidetoContrastMedia.aspx. Accessed September 5, 2010.
8. Visipaque [package insert]. Princeton, NJ: GE Healthcare Inc. (manufactured by GE Healthcare Ireland; Cork, Ireland); May 2008.
9. Ioxaglate. Drugdex Evaluations Micromedex. www.thomsonhc.com. Accessed May 3, 2010 (access available only to subscribers).
10. Diatrizoate. Drugdex Evaluations Micromedex. www.thomsonhc.com. Accessed May 3, 2010 (access available only to subscribers).

11. Omnipaque [package insert]. Princeton, NJ: GE Healthcare Inc (manufactured by GE Healthcare Ireland; Cork, Ireland); May 2008.
12. American College of Radiology. Contrast media in children. In: ACR Manual on Contrast Media, version 7, 2010. www.acr.org/SecondaryMainMenuCategories/quality_safety/contrast_manual/FullManual.aspx#page=7. Accessed September 5, 2010.
13. Jensen SC, Peppers MP. Pharmacodynamics of radiopaque contrast media. In: Jensen SC, Peppers MP, eds. *Pharmacology and Drug Administration for Imaging Technologists.* 2nd ed. St Louis: Mosby Elsevier; 2006:81–99.
14. Webb JAW. Prevention of acute reactions. In: Thomsen HS, Webb JAW, eds. *Medical Radiology Diagnostic Imaging: Contrast Media Safety Issues and ESUR Guidelines.* 2nd ed. Berlin, Heidelberg: Springer-Verlag; 2009:43–51.
15. Thrall JH. Adverse reactions to contrast media: etiology, incidence, treatment, and prevention. In: Swanson DP, Chilton HM, Thrall JH, eds. *Pharmaceuticals in Medical Imaging.* New York: Macmillan; 1990:253–77.
16. Briguori C, Tavano D, Colombo A. Contrast agent-associated nephrotoxicity. *Prog Cardiovasc Dis.* 2003;45:493–503.
17. Thomsen HS. Contrast medium-induced nephropathy. In: Thomsen HS, Webb JAW, eds. *Medical Radiology Diagnostic Imaging: Contrast Media Safety Issues and ESUR Guidelines.* 2nd ed. Berlin, Heidelberg: Springer-Verlag; 2009:63–80.
18. Solomon R, Deray G. How to prevent contrast-induced nephropathy and manage risk patients: practical recommendations. *Kidney Int Suppl.* 2006;69:S51–53.
19. Katayama H, Yamaguchi K, Kozuka T, et al. Adverse reactions to ionic and non-ionic contrast media. *Radiology.* 1990;175:621–8.
20. Intrathecal injection of ionic contrast media may be fatal. *ISMP Medication Safety Alert!* (November 27, 2003). www.ismp.org/newsletters/acutecare/articles/20031127.asp. Accessed August 15, 2010.
21. Marcos SK. Interactions with other drugs and clinical tests. In: Thomsen HS, Webb JAW, eds. *Medical Radiology Diagnostic Imaging: Contrast Media Safety Issues and ESUR Guidelines.* 2nd ed. Berlin, Heidelberg: Springer-Verlag; 2009:107–13.
22. Webb JAW. Non-insulin-dependent diabetes and contrast media. In: Thomsen HS, Webb JAW, eds. *Medical Radiology Diagnostic Imaging: Contrast Media Safety Issues and ESUR Guidelines.* 2nd ed. Berlin, Heidelberg: Springer-Verlag; 2009:87–92.
23. Jensen SC, Peppers MP. Drug classifications. In: Jensen SC, Peppers MP, eds. *Pharmacology and Drug Administration for Imaging Technologists.* 2nd ed. St Louis: Mosby Elsevier; 2006:54–63.
24. Kowalsky RJ, Falen SW. Thyroid. In: Kowalsky RJ, Falen SW, eds. *Radiopharmaceuticals in Nuclear Pharmacy and Nuclear Medicine.* 2nd ed. Washington, DC: American Pharmacists Association; 2004:495–513.
25. Swanson DP, Halpert RD. Gastrointestinal contrast media: barium sulfate and water-soluble iodinated agents. In: Swanson DP, Chilton HM, Thrall JH, eds. *Pharmaceuticals in Medical Imaging.* New York: Macmillan; 1990:155–83.
26. Morcos SK. Barium preparations: safety issues. In: Thomsen HS, Webb JAW, eds. *Medical Radiology Diagnostic Imaging: Contrast Media Safety Issues and ESUR Guidelines.* 2nd ed. Berlin, Heidelberg: Springer-Verlag; 2009:223–6.
27. Barium. Drugdex Evaluations Micromedex. www.thomsonhc.com. Accessed September 5, 2010 (access available only to subscribers).

28. Barosperse [package insert]. St Louis: Mallinckrodt; September 2006.
29. Prepcat [package insert]. St Louis: Mallinckrodt; April 2006.
30. Javors BR, Applbaum Y, Gerard P. Severe allergic reaction: an unusual complication of barium enema. *Gastrointest Radiol.* 1984;9:357–8.
31. Katsanoulas C, Passakiotou M, Mouloudi E, et al. Severe barium sulphate aspiration: a report of two cases and review of the literature. *Signa Vitae.* 2007;2:25–8. www.signavitae.com/articles/case-reports/22-severe-barium-sulphate-aspiration-a-report-of-two-cases-and-review-of-the-literature. Accessed September 5, 2010.
32. Gastrografin [package insert]. Princeton, NJ: Bracco Diagnostics; September 2007.
33. Fan ST, Lau WY, Yip WC, et al. Limitations and dangers of gastrografin swallow after esophageal and upper gastric operations. *Am J Surg.* 1988;155:495–7.

CHAPTER 5

Review of Imaging Procedures Using Nuclear Medicine and Positron Emission Tomography

Brian Schumer

Nuclear medicine is a diagnostic imaging modality that uses low levels of radioactive material to trace physiologic processes within the body. In contrast to x-ray imaging, in which ionizing radiation is passed through the body from an external source, the radioactive material used in nuclear medicine is placed inside the patient's body and allowed to circulate. Nuclear medicine also differs from magnetic resonance imaging (MRI) and ultrasound imaging, which do not use ionizing radiation. All diagnostic imaging modalities show anatomic structure to varying degrees, but x-ray, MRI, and ultrasound imaging have limited ability to identify and quantify the functional capacity of the organs and organ systems being imaged. The key advantage of nuclear imaging is its ability to provide anatomic information while also providing fairly detailed information about organ function. Nuclear medicine continues to evolve, with growing emphasis on positron emission tomography (PET), a nuclear medicine specialty that provides greater anatomic detail along with a strong interpretation of various physiologic processes that occur within the body.

Radiation in Nature

Radiation is all around us. Naturally occurring radiation is present in the soil, our food, the air we breathe, and even our own bodies. Natural radiation levels may differ significantly by location. For example, residents of higher altitudes (e.g., Colorado) are exposed to higher levels of cosmic radiation from outer space than are residents of locations closer to sea level.[1] People who happen to live in Cornwall or Aberdeenshire in the United Kingdom experience an unusually high level of radon exposure. Radon is a decay product of uranium that is present in ore-bearing rocks around the world. Radon seeps from these rocks into the water, soil, and atmosphere, exposing inhabitants to high concentrations of this gaseous element. The average radiation exposure of someone living in the United States is about 300 mrem per year, and two-thirds of this exposure can be attributed to radon. Another 60 mrem can be attributed to manmade sources of radiation such as those used in commercial and medical industries.

Despite the abundance of radioactive sources in the earth, the atmosphere, and outer space, none of this natural radiation possesses the qualities considered ideal for treating and imaging patients. The natural isotopes are too difficult to obtain and are unsafe for human administration. For example, uranium 238 (^{238}U) has a half-life of about 4.47 billion years and decays by emitting an alpha particle, the most damaging type of radioactive decay. An isotope with a much shorter half-life and lower-energy gamma decay would be safer for human use.

Early Use of Radionuclides

Although research on radioactivity began in the 1800s, it is hard to pinpoint the birth of nuclear medicine. Many people consider the most significant milestone in nuclear medicine to be the discovery of artificially produced isotopes in 1934 by Frederic Joliot and Irene Joliot-Curie. They used a polonium source to bombard an aluminum target with alpha particles. When they removed the polonium source, they noticed that the target continued to emit radiation. The aluminum had transformed into a new element that was now radioactive. The new element was phosphorus 30 (^{30}P), one of the first artificially made radionuclides.[2] Two years later, in 1936, John H. Lawrence used phosphorus 32 (^{32}P) to treat leukemia, marking the first time an artificial radionuclide was used therapeutically. In 1946, Samuel M. Seidlin published an article in the *Journal of the American Medical Association* that would change the course of nuclear medicine and help usher in its widespread clinical use in the 1950s. The article described how radioiodine (^{131}I) was successfully used to cure thyroid cancer. In 1950, Abbott Laboratories marketed the first commercial radiopharmaceutical, ^{131}I-human serum albumin (RISA). In 1951, ^{131}I-sodium iodide became the first FDA-approved radiopharmaceutical. The use of ^{131}I expanded from the treatment of thyroid cancer to include imaging of the thyroid gland, evaluation of its function, and treatment of hyperthyroidism.

The rapid growth and widespread use of nuclear medicine led to a flurry of research and the development of new radionuclides and radiopharmaceuticals. Among these was technetium 99m (^{99m}Tc), one of the most important discoveries in the history of nuclear medicine. This valuable radioisotope was nearly overlooked when it was discovered as a trace contaminant during the production of iodine 132 from tellurium 132. Walter Tucker and Margaret Greene found that technetium was generated from its parent isotope, molybdenum 99, and that it displayed decay characteristics and a parent–daughter relationship similar to that of tellurium and iodine. At the U.S. Department of Energy's Brookhaven National Laboratory, Tucker and Greene developed the first molybdenum 99–technetium 99m (^{99}Mo–^{99m}Tc) generator. Powell Richards, in charge of isotope production at Brookhaven, realized the potential of ^{99m}Tc and began promoting it among other medical professionals.

^{99m}Tc Generator Systems and Radiopharmaceutical Kits

The short half-life of ^{99m}Tc (6 hours) is long enough to allow time for medical procedures but short enough that the isotope is quickly eliminated from the patient. Its low-energy gamma photon (140 keV) allows it to be imaged easily without damaging body tissue with radiation. Furthermore, ^{99}Mo has a long enough half-life (66 hours) to allow it to be shipped all over the world. A generator system using the parent isotope ^{99}Mo made ^{99m}Tc easily accessible to any local market.

^{99m}Tc generator systems consist of an alumina anion-exchange column bound with ^{99}Mo. The column is placed in a lead shield with tubing attached to each end. A vial of normal saline (0.9% sodium chloride) is placed at one end of the tube, while an evacuated vial is placed at the other end. As the saline solution is pulled across the column, ^{99m}Tc is washed off with the saline while the ^{99}Mo remains tightly bound to the alumina column. This produces radioactive saline that consists almost entirely of ^{99m}Tc. This radioactive saline, or "tech," can then be used to compound radiopharmaceutical kits. With its low energy level and short half-life, ^{99m}Tc quickly became the ideal radionuclide for nuclear medicine studies.[3]

Unfortunately, ^{99m}Tc itself had limited applications for imaging, given its natural distribution in the GI tract, the thyroid, and the salivary glands and retention in the blood pool. However, the technetium molecule lends itself to various radiolabeling reactions that allow the radioactive isotope to be attached to different molecules that behave in certain ways within the body. By simply attaching a radioactive isotope like ^{99m}Tc, it is possible to make a molecule radioactive and, with camera technology, to watch the movement of the molecule through the body. These radiolabeled products are referred to as "kits." Each kit is designed to locate to a different organ of the body, allowing the imaging of that organ and evaluation of its function. The molecule that is bound to the ^{99m}Tc is referred to as a ligand. The ligand mimics specific physiologic processes, making it possible to image and evaluate them. For example, diphosphonates (^{99m}Tc-MDP, ^{99m}Tc-HDP) are used to image bones. Phosphates are absorbed by all bone, but to varying degrees. Diseased or damaged bone is constantly involved in osteoblastic activity as the body tries to repair and build the bone; these areas absorb more phosphate than others. Using ^{99m}Tc attached to a diphosphonate molecule will show these areas as "hot spots" on the image, or areas of increased radioactivity. To ensure that no pharmacologic effect is observed, very small amounts of ligand are used. The goal is to image the body's natural processes, not to modify how the natural processes occur.[4]

A radiopharmaceutical kit consists of a sterile reaction vial containing a ligand and a reducing agent, typically stannous chloride. Other ingredients may include buffers, stabilizers, and dispersing agents. Because the stannous ion is easily oxidized, the vial is usually purged of oxygen with nitrogen or another inert gas. Kit preparation varies depending on the particular radiopharmaceutical being prepared. In general, ^{99m}Tc is added using aseptic technique and then the kit is brought to a specific volume with normal saline to give a desired concentration. Most kits require an incubation period to allow for the "tagging" process to occur before doses are withdrawn. Some kits require heating to facilitate the tagging process. Since the 1970s, many radiopharmaceutical kit formulations have been produced. This has allowed the visualization of a number of internal organs and organ systems, including the liver, spleen, and GI tract, and the localization of brain tumors. The ability to diagnose heart disease followed in the 1980s, as well as the use of digital computers to enhance processing of the images.

PET Imaging

PET is a type of nuclear medicine imaging that offers very detailed information about the physiology of various organ systems. The functional nature of PET allows data processing and evaluation at the cellular level. With the use of a cyclotron, short-lived radioisotopes of basic organic elements such as carbon (^{11}C), nitrogen (^{13}N), oxygen (^{15}O), and fluorine (^{18}F) can be produced. These radioactive isotopes can then be tagged to common organic molecules found in the body so that images of specific body processes or organ systems can be obtained. The basis of PET is the positron, a positively charged beta particle emitted from a neutron-poor radionuclide. The positrons interact with electrons through annihilation, resulting in two 511-keV gamma rays traveling in opposite directions. PET cameras can detect these opposing events. If both gamma rays are not detected directly opposite each other, then the event is not counted.

Large particle accelerators called cyclotrons are used to produce PET radioisotopes. A cyclotron consists of two dipole magnets—called Dees for their D shape—designed to create a semicircular region of uniform magnetic field. An oscillating voltage is applied to the Dees to produce an electrical field in the gap between the two magnets. When a charged particle is injected into the magnetic field, it traces the semicircular path of the Dees and is accelerated each time it passes the electrical field between the magnets until it is propelled from the current toward an awaiting target.[4]

Radiopharmaceutical Compounding

Radiopharmaceuticals are compounded using aseptic technique in a controlled environment. Historically, many large hospitals had in-house radiopharmacies where they could compound kits and draw doses on site. Most other hospitals, outpatient clinics, and cardiology offices would typically order doses from a centralized pharmacy that would deliver them daily. In 2004, the first set of standards for sterile compounding was published by the United States Pharmacopeia.[5] Commonly referred to as "USP 797," this document provided strict guidance regarding the environment and method in which sterile drugs were to be compounded. Because radiopharmaceuticals are primarily injected intravenously, their preparation falls under these standards. Many institutions have had to rethink how to meet their radiopharmaceutical needs. In view of the high cost of cleanrooms and ISO class 5 devices, many institutions have moved toward ordering unit doses from centralized pharmacies.

Imaging Equipment

Once a radiopharmaceutical has been injected into the patient, a way of quantifying the data and creating an image is needed. Early instruments used for the detection of radiation in the body were simply handheld Geiger-Müller counters and scintillation probes. These allowed for overall counting of radioactivity in the body but did not allow for spatial localization. In 1950, Benedict Cassen invented the rectilinear scanner. This device used a single photon detector that moved laterally across the body, detecting and analyzing emitted radiation to build an image line by line. In 1952, Hal Anger developed the first gamma camera. It consisted of a pinhole camera with a sodium iodide crystal as the detector and a photographic plate. This camera was capable of imaging entire organs at once, but it still took an hour or more to obtain them. Anger continued to work on the gamma camera and, in 1956, developed a concept still used in gamma cameras today. This camera consisted of a 4-inch sodium iodide crystal as the scintillator coupled with seven closely packed photomultiplier tubes (PMTs). A scintillator, in this case the sodium iodide crystal, is a transparent material that converts energy lost by ionization into a pulse of light. The amount of light produced is proportional to the energy deposited by the incident. When the crystal absorbs a gamma ray, the scintillation light created is spread across the PMTs, which then convert the light to an electrical signal and amplify it. Centroiding logic ("Anger" logic) calculates the exact position of each event within the crystal, allowing an image to be constructed.[6]

To gain spatial resolution, collimators are placed directly in front of the scintillation crystal. A collimator is a lead disk with thousands of holes drilled through it, which will limit crystal detection to only those photons entering the collimator directly above a particular hole. Any photon emitted from the patient outside the angle of view will be absorbed by the lead and will not be counted. Without the collimator, a photon could hit the crystal at any point on its surface, making it impossible to determine the photon's point of origin in the body. A downside of the use of collimators is that less than 1% of photons reach the camera. This leads to poor sensitivity of the image.

With the development of computed tomography (CT), we have seen great improvements in camera technology and the quality of images. A single-photon emission computed tomography (SPECT) camera now has one to three detectors that rotate around the patient, collecting two-dimensional images at points 360° around the patient. Computer reconstruction displays the information in three planes: transverse, sagittal, and coronal. Algorithms are then capable of constructing a three-dimensional picture from many two-dimensional ones. SPECT imaging has a much greater target-to-nontarget ratio than traditional planar imaging. The foreground and background activity present in planar imaging is virtually eliminated in the SPECT reconstruction process.

PET imaging is based on the presence of a positron-emitting radionuclide producing two 511-keV annihilation photons traveling in opposite directions. A ring of detectors is used to pick up these associated photons. Because only coincident photons directly opposing each other are detected, there is no need for a collimator. All other events will be disregarded. With no need for a collimator, the sensitivity of PET imaging is increased significantly over planar or SPECT cameras. Further advances in imaging have combined multiple modalities, such as PET/CT and PET/MRI, in which the detailed functional information of PET is combined with the superior structural images of CT and MRI. The images can be superimposed on each other for an impeccable picture of the body's organs.

Diagnostic Imaging Agents

Although early nuclear medicine studies focused on the treatment and imaging of the thyroid, this specialty quickly expanded to include imaging studies of almost every organ in the body. The localization of radiopharmaceuticals in different organs is based on cellular function and physiology, giving nuclear medicine the ability to evaluate organ function and disease processes. Therefore, nuclear medicine can often identify problems earlier than can other imaging modalities that rely solely on physical changes in anatomic structure. Organ systems and conditions that can be studied using nuclear medicine procedures are discussed briefly below.

Adrenal Gland

The adrenal glands are situated above each kidney and normally weigh about 5 grams. In conditions of excess adrenocorticotrophic hormone (ACTH), the gland may enlarge to as much as 20 grams. It is a two-part structure, consisting of the outer cortex and the inner medulla. The adrenal cortex produces three major types of steroid hormones: mineralocorticoids, glucocorticoids, and androgens. When secreted in excess, the adrenocortical hormones produce distinct signs and symptoms. Epinephrine is the primary catecholamine hormone secreted by the adrenal medulla. Before performing nuclear medicine imaging, it is essential to distinguish adrenocortical dysfunction from sympathomedullary dysfunction. The imaging agent of choice for adrenocortical scintigraphy is ^{131}I-6 beta-iodomethyl-norcholesterol (NP-59), which localizes in the cortex as a result of the transport and receptor systems for serum cholesterol bound to low-density lipoprotein (LDL). Increases in ACTH result in increased radiocholesterol uptake.[7] The most common indication for adrenocortical scintigraphy is hypercortisolism, or Cushing's syndrome. Adrenomedullary scintigraphy is useful in the management of patients with functional adrenergic tumors, including paragangliomas, neuroblastomas, and pheochromocytomas. The imaging agent of choice for these disorders is ^{123}I- or ^{131}I-meta-iodobenzylguanidine (MIBG). MIBG should not be used in a screening procedure for pheochromocytoma; it should be used only after biochemical tests suggest the diagnosis. Many centers use CT first to evaluate the adrenals. If a mass is present, then further workup is necessary before surgery. MIBG is particularly useful for scanning the entire body for metastatic disease and extra-adrenal tumors.

Brain and Cerebrospinal Fluid

Nuclear medicine studies for brain imaging focus on blood perfusion of the brain. The blood–brain barrier selectively prevents certain substances from crossing over into the brain matter. Early brain imaging agents were nonlipophilic agents that were unable to cross the blood–brain barrier; therefore, they were useful only for evaluating blood flow to the skull. These agents could only detect whether blood was leaking out of the vessels, as in aneurysm or head trauma. With the development of lipophilic tracers that were able to cross into the brain tissue, information about the functional capacity of brain tissue could be obtained. These agents include ^{99m}Tc-exametazime (Ceretec [GE Healthcare]) and ^{99m}Tc-bicisate (Neurolite [Lantheus]).

Clinical indications for these brain perfusion imaging agents include aid in the detection of stroke, brain tumor recurrence, brain death, seizure focus, and transient ischemic attack (TIA) and evaluation of brain injury and perfusion patterns, Alzheimer's disease, and other causes of dementia. A normal scan will show uniform uptake of the radiopharmaceutical in the brain tissue, indicating appropriate blood flow through the brain. In instances of stroke or TIA, the image reveals areas of regional blood perfusion deficiency. In the case of brain death, no perfusion of the brain is seen. An active seizure focus is indicated by an increase in blood flow to the site in comparison with surrounding brain tissue.

SPECT imaging provides spatial data for brain imaging. PET imaging plays an important role by enabling brain metabolism studies with the use of fludeoxyglucose F 18 injection (^{18}F-FDG). Clinical applications for PET imaging include the evaluation of epilepsy, movement disorders, cerebrovascular disease, and dementia.[8]

Nuclear medicine studies of cerebrospinal fluid, the colorless, clear liquid that surrounds and protects the brain and spinal cord, include cisternography and leakage studies. Cisternography provides information regarding the formation, movement, and resorption of the cerebrospinal fluid in the body. Leakage studies determine where the fluid may be leaking from the compartment it usually occupies.

^{111}In-pentetate (^{111}In-DTPA) is the radiopharmaceutical used in these imaging studies.

Cancer

Nuclear medicine studies use ^{67}Ga for tumor imaging in Hodgkin's and non-Hodgkin's lymphoma. Nuclear medicine also uses radiolabeled antibodies for diagnostic imaging of certain cancers. ^{111}In-capromab pendetide (ProstaScint [Cytogen]) is a monoclonal antibody that binds to prostate-specific antigen (PSA), which is found in high concentrations in patients with prostate cancer. This agent is indicated for newly diagnosed patients thought to be at high risk for pelvic lymph node metastatic disease and for patients who have had their prostate removed and show no evidence of metastatic disease but have a rising PSA level and high clinical suspicion of metastatic disease.

Cardiac

Myocardial perfusion imaging—the most widely used nuclear medicine study—offers cardiologists a quick, inexpensive, and noninvasive test of blood flow and cell viability in the heart. Thallium 201 (^{201}Tl) was the first radiopharmaceutical used for myocardial imaging and is still widely used today. ^{201}Tl behaves much like K^+, taking advantage of free access to myocardial cells via the Na^+-K^+ ATPase pump. Images taken soon after injection reflect capillary blood flow through the heart. After uptake, ^{201}Tl demonstrates redistribution, meaning it moves freely between the myocardial cells and the blood pool. Several hours after injection, the cellular ^{201}Tl and the ^{201}Tl in the blood pool reach equilibrium, reflecting regional blood volume. In normal perfusion studies, the early blood flow images and the later regional blood volume images are similar. The unique properties of ^{201}Tl imaging are the basis of the stress–redistribution tests used to evaluate coronary artery disease. Patients are "stressed" for the early image, meaning they achieve 80% of their maximum heart rate by means of treadmill exercise or pharmacologic stress agents. "Cold" spots (areas of decreased activity) reflect areas of decreased blood flow due to either blockage of vessels in that area or lack of viable cells. A "rest" image is taken later. If the cold spots fill in, this represents ischemia. If they continue to lack isotope activity, the cells are no longer viable (infarct).

More recently, as a result of the favorable imaging characteristics of ^{99m}Tc, the agents ^{99m}Tc-sestamibi (Cardiolite [Lantheus]) and ^{99m}Tc-tetrofosmin (Myoview [GE Healthcare]) have allowed higher resolution and more detailed images. Rather than demonstrating redistribution as does ^{201}Tl, these lipophilic compounds are trapped in the myocardium. The imaging concept is similar, but because of their higher administered doses, higher photoenergy emissions (140 keV versus 69 to 83 keV), and distinct photopeak, these agents produce superior images on modern-day cameras.

The use of PET agents for cardiac perfusion studies is increasing, especially with the advent of the ^{82}Rb generator. Because of the high cost of the generator delivery system, the use of this agent still is generally limited to clinics and hospitals that perform a high volume of myocardial perfusion studies.

Multiple gated acquisition (MUGA) cardiac imaging enables the identification of cardiac wall motion abnormalities and left ventricular ejection fraction through the use of red blood cells (RBCs) obtained from the patient, radiolabeled with ^{99m}Tc, and reinjected prior to imaging. Indications for MUGA are the staging of congestive heart failure, preoperative cardiac evaluation, and cardiac transplant assessment.

Gastrointestinal

Gastric emptying studies are used to quantitatively and qualitatively assess gastric motility.[8] Depending on the isotope used, either liquid or solid gastric emptying can be evaluated. Studies in adults are more commonly performed with solids; ^{99m}Tc-sulfur colloid is added to eggs, oatmeal, or chicken liver, which the patient eats prior to imaging. Liquid gastric emptying studies can be performed using ^{111}In-DTPA mixed in water, milk, or juice; because of the limited availability of this isotope, most institutions perform only solid gastric emptying imaging. For pediatric patients unable to ingest a solid meal, ^{99m}Tc-sulfur colloid is mixed with formula. Images are obtained over a period of time, with regions of interest set around the stomach. Changes in the radioactivity counts over time are monitored to determine the percentage of emptying. In patients with delayed gastric emptying, gastric reflux and aspiration studies may be performed to determine whether the delay in emptying is contributing to either of these conditions.

Nuclear medicine imaging can be used to confirm and localize Meckel's diverticulum, a congenital defect in the lower GI tract. A small percentage of Meckel's diverticula contain gastric mucosa that can secrete acid and lead to damage to the lower GI tract. ^{99m}Tc-sodium pertechnetate is normally taken up by gastric mucosa in the stomach and will also be taken up by gastric mucosa in the diverticulum.

Nuclear medicine is also used to identify GI bleeding by reinjecting the patient's ^{99m}Tc-labeled RBCs. If the patient is bleeding into the GI tract, the radiolabeled RBCs will leak into the GI tract and show up on the images as a focal accumulation of radioactivity in the GI lumen. The benefit of this procedure is that it is possible to evaluate intermittent GI bleeding because imaging can be performed over extended periods of time.

Hepatobiliary

The hepatobiliary system consists of the hepatocytes in the liver, the gallbladder, and the associated system of ducts that connect each component and eventually associate with the GI tract via the small intestine. The function of this system is to produce, store, and release bile. Nuclear medicine studies are performed to evaluate right upper quadrant pain and recurrent jaundice, diagnose acute cholecystitis and differentiate acute from chronic cholecystitis, detect biliary leaks after surgery, differentiate between biliary atresia and neonatal hepatitis, and determine gallbladder ejection fraction. The radiopharmaceuticals used for hepatobiliary system indications work by following the path of bile through the organ system. ^{99m}Tc-disofenin (Hepatolite [Pharmalucence]) and ^{99m}Tc-mebrofenin (Choletec [Bracco]) are the radiopharmaceuticals used for imaging. The images obtained can provide functional information on the liver by assessing the rate of radiopharmaceutical uptake by the hepatocytes, the first step in bile formation. The biliary ejection fraction, a measurement of the amount of bile, may be obtained to further aid in diagnosis. An ejection fraction greater than 35% is normal, whereas a value less than 35% suggests defective gallbladder contraction that could be due to cholecystitis or other abnormalities.[8]

Sometimes nonradiopharmaceuticals are needed to aid in the nuclear medicine study. A synthetic version of the endogenous substance cholecystokinin may be used to cause contraction of the gallbladder for determination of the ejection fraction. Also, morphine may be used if no gallbladder is seen on the images 1 hour after injection of the radiopharmaceutical. If the gallbladder is not seen after the morphine injection, this indicates acute cholecystitis possibly due to an obstruction within the biliary system. If the gallbladder is seen after the morphine injection, then the diagnosis most likely is chronic cholecystitis due to a thickened or fibrotic gallbladder wall that causes the gallbladder to eject bile inefficiently.

Infection

Infections are a major, costly problem in medical care. To treat infections quickly and effectively, a rapid diagnosis is needed. Nuclear medicine uses radiolabeled white blood cells (WBCs) to locate the site of infection, since WBCs migrate to infectious processes in the body. A sample of the patient's blood is removed and the WBCs are isolated and radiolabeled using either ^{111}In-oxine or ^{99m}Tc-exametazime (Ceretec). After reinjection into the patient, the white cells migrate to the site of infection, resulting in a focal accumulation of activity at the site. WBC labeling is particularly useful in abdominal infections, is not so useful in chest infections, and gives mixed results in bone infections. Nuclear medicine imaging using labeled WBCs is also good for detecting ulcerative colitis and Crohn's disease. ^{67}Ga-citrate can also be used for imaging infection, but it is more useful in patients with chronic infectious processes. Clinical applications for ^{67}Ga-citrate are fever of unknown origin, sarcoidosis, and AIDS-related infections.

Lung

Nuclear imaging is used to evaluate two distinct aspects of lung function: perfusion and ventilation. ^{99m}Tc-macroaggregated albumin (MAA) is used to assess blood flow in the lung. It lodges in the capillaries to create a detailed map of blood flow through the organ. It is often used in patients with possible pulmonary embolism and to evaluate perfusion changes in emphysema, chronic bronchitis, asthma, and inflammatory disease.[4] For ventilation studies, ^{133}Xe gas or aerosolized ^{99m}Tc-DTPA is commonly used. After the patient inhales the radioactive material, an image of the lungs' ventilation capacity and capability can be obtained.

Lymphoscintigraphy and Sentinel Node Mapping

The lymphatic system collects and returns interstitial fluid to help maintain fluid balance in the body, produces lymphocytes, and absorbs lipids from the intestines and moves them to the blood. This system includes many organs as well as an extensive network of vessels that drain lymph from all over the body. Lymph nodes are a network of tissue containing macrophages and phagocytes that remove foreign material, debris, and bacteria from lymph. Because the lymphatic system is so widespread in the body, it plays an important role in the metastasis of some cancers. When a patient has a tumor, lymph nodes surrounding the tumor may be removed or biopsied to reveal whether the cancer has spread from its origin.

One method of accurately identifying the primary lymph node to which a tumor bed will drain is called sentinel node mapping or lymphoscintigraphy. The first lymph node in the chain of lymph nodes that drains a given area of the body is called the sentinel node. During surgical removal of certain cancers, removal and biopsy of nearby lymph nodes will provide information on the likelihood of spread of the disease from the primary tumor bed. In many cases, this is an extensive undertaking, as it is difficult to know which lymph node is involved in the drainage from the tumor site. Nuclear medicine imaging allows identification of the sentinel node through watching the migration of a radiolabeled pharmaceutical from an injection site near the primary tumor. Once the tracer is taken up, imaging can be performed to locate the sentinel node for surgical removal and biopsy. If the sentinel node is cancerous, it can be deduced that the cancer has spread from the primary tumor site, and treatment will be tailored for metastatic disease rather than for localized disease.

The radiopharmaceutical used for this procedure is ^{99m}Tc-sulfur colloid, an insoluble particulate that is picked up by the lymphatic system and carried to the node chain. ^{99m}Tc-sulfur colloid is injected intradermally into the area surrounding the tumor site, and sufficient time is allowed for the tracer to move through the lymphatic channels into the sentinel node prior to surgery. During surgery, a small gamma probe can be used to easily identify a "hot" node that will then be removed for biopsy. Lymphoscintigraphy is most commonly used in patients with breast cancer and dermatologic cancers such as melanoma.

Renal

The kidneys are the waste removal organs of the body. Glomerular filtration and active tubular secretion are the kidney's main mechanisms of waste removal. Nuclear medicine studies can be used to evaluate renal function, as the agents themselves will follow one of the two normal excretion pathways. Glomerular filtration is the removal of water and dissolved substances from the blood. To evaluate glomerular filtration, ^{99m}Tc-DTPA or ^{125}I-iothalamate (Glofil-125 [IsoTex Diagnostics]) is used, since these agents are excreted by the glomerular filtration pathway. Tubular reabsorption occurs when substances are returned to the blood as they pass through the tubules and loop of Henle in the nephron. Nonfiltered substances can be removed by the kidneys through tubular secretion. ^{99m}Tc-mertiatide, also referred to as ^{99m}Tc-MAG-3, is excreted through tubular secretion; it has become the agent most commonly used for renal imaging. Often, diuretics or angiotensin-converting enzyme (ACE) inhibitors are administered during the studies to aid in the evaluation or to enhance the amount of information obtained by altering the physiologic process being studied. Clinical indications for these types of studies include renal artery stenosis, renovascular hypertension, renal transplant assessment, and posttransplant rejection.

^{99m}Tc-succimer, also called ^{99m}Tc-DMSA, is classified as a renal morphology agent. It is used to assess the renal parenchyma without the influence of the collecting system's activity. Such agents are retained in the kidney for extended periods and thus provide information on the shape and size of the kidney and identify renal masses and scarring that may affect kidney function.

Reticuloendothelial

The reticuloendothelial system (RES) comprises the liver, spleen, and bone marrow. The function of the RES is to remove and phagocytize foreign substances, cellular debris, and pathogens from the blood. The liver has two major types of cells—the hepatocytes, which produce bile, and Kupffer's cells, which scavenge for foreign material. The Kupffer's cells are the RES cells of the liver. The spleen, the largest lymphatic organ in the body, is the part of the RES responsible for removing abnormal blood components. The bone marrow found in large bones produces and stores blood components. Clinical applications for RES imaging include differential diagnosis for liver masses; diagnostic correlation with other modalities such as CT, ultrasound, and MRI; and diagnosis of Budd-Chiari syndrome. The radiopharmaceutical that is phagocytized by RES cells is ^{99m}Tc-sulfur colloid, an insoluble particulate. After IV administration, the particles are rapidly cleared from the circulation by the phagocytic activity of the RES cells. Uptake patterns of the tracer indicate different diseases. "Hot" spots in the liver can indicate Budd-Chiari syndrome, whereas "cold" spots indicate metastatic disease, cysts, abscesses, or cirrhosis. This imaging procedure also provides some information about the functional capacity of the liver. In some cases, a "colloid shift" can be seen, in which there is increased colloid uptake by other RES tissue as a result of severe liver disease.

Skeletal

Skeletal imaging, one of the most important and most frequently used nuclear medicine procedures, is used most often for the evaluation of metastatic disease, infection, and traumatic injury. Unlike standard x-ray imaging, in which only significant changes in bone density and structure can be noticed, radiolabeled bone agents have high sensitivity for revealing even the smallest changes in skeletal cell remodeling. Bone tissue is active and constantly changing, and ligands designed to participate in these processes can be used to carry a radioisotope to the region of interest.[7] For decades, compounds containing phosphate groups have been used to image the bone remodeling process, as phosphate is a key component in the structure of bone tissue. ^{99m}Tc-labeled methylene diphosphonate (^{99m}Tc-MDP) and hydroxymethylene diphosphonate (^{99m}Tc-HDP) are the current agents of choice. Their high sensitivity, ready availability, reasonable cost, and ability to scan the entire skeleton make them a popular choice despite technologic advances in MRI, CT, and PET imaging. The major disadvantage is their low specificity. Any alteration in bone remodeling will be seen on a bone scan but may not be due to a particular disease process of concern. For example, uptake in the joints is not uncommon, especially in older patients who may have excessive remodeling due to stress or because of arthritic changes in the joints. This most likely is not diagnostic if the patient is being evaluated for metastatic spread of cancer to the bone. Unfortunately, the appearance of the scan would be similar, so an understanding of the patient's clinical status is needed for interpretation of the results.

Thyroid

The thyroid gland is a butterfly-shaped organ with two lateral lobes on either side of the thyroid cartilage. The gland of an average adult normally weighs 15 to 20 grams, but the appearance varies from patient to patient. The lateral lobes typically measure 4 to 5 cm from superior to inferior pole and are 1.5 to 2 cm wide. The right lobe is often larger than the left.[7] Nuclear medicine procedures can be used to diagnose a wide array of thyroid diseases including hyperthyroidism, thyroiditis, Graves' disease, and thyroid nodules. Both ^{99m}Tc-sodium pertechnetate and ^{123}I-sodium iodide are used to image the thyroid. A benefit of using the radioactive iodine compound is that the iodine will be taken up and organified in the thyroid gland and synthesized into thyroid hormone just as nonradioactive iodine would be. ^{99m}Tc-sodium pertechnetate, on the other hand, is picked up by the same transporter because of its size, but once inside the gland it cannot participate in the hormone synthesis pathway and will eventually wash out of the gland. Because of this, ^{123}I-sodium iodide is more accurate for evaluating thyroid function, whereas ^{99m}Tc-sodium pertechnetate is generally used as an anatomic imaging agent. ^{131}I-sodium iodide can also be used for functional determination and imaging, but it is not preferred because of its longer half-life (8.04 days) and beta particle emissions. ^{131}I-sodium iodide is usually reserved for treatment of thyroid disorders, most notably Graves' disease, hyperthyroidism, and thyroid cancer.[2]

Therapeutic Imaging Agents

Although this book focuses on diagnostic imaging, nuclear medicine can also be used for therapeutic applications, in which the inherent qualities of radiation are used to treat a disease rather than to diagnose it. Since many of the isotopes used for therapeutic purposes also possess radioactive emissions that can be imaged using traditional methods, it is possible to not only treat certain diseases but to identify where the disease is located and verify that all areas of disease have uptake of the tracer and therefore are receiving some level of therapeutic benefit. Some of the more common therapeutic radiopharmaceutical applications are summarized below.

Thyroid

Nuclear medicine therapy for the thyroid is indicated for hyperthyroidism and thyroid cancer. The radioisotope of choice is ^{131}I, as it will be taken up by thyroid tissue but the presence of beta emissions can provide therapeutic benefit. The ^{131}I beta emissions cause fibrosis and destruction of the thyroid tissue, leading to a decrease in the functional portion of the thyroid. A major benefit of this type of therapy is that the beta radiation will travel only a short distance (~1 mm) in tissue and will cause damage that is essentially confined to the thyroid gland. In the treatment of hyperthyroidism, the goal is to decrease overfunctioning tissue while still maintaining viable tissue that will produce endogenous thyroid hormone; this condition, euthyroidism, is the desired outcome of therapy in most patients. However, it is possible to undertreat the patient (resulting in continued hyperthyroidism) or overtreat the patient (resulting in hypothyroidism), so careful determination of thyroid function and of accurate therapeutic doses is important. For thyroid cancer, the standard treatment in most institutions is surgical removal of the thyroid gland. After surgery, high-dose ^{131}I-sodium iodide is administered to try to ablate any residual tissue that remains in the body, either at the site of surgery or in metastatic lesions.

Bone Pain Palliation

Bone pain palliation is needed when a primary cancer has metastasized to the bone and begun growing there, causing pain through a variety of mechanisms. Treatment options for alleviating bone pain include radiation therapy, surgery, hormonal therapy, chemotherapy, pain medication, and radiopharmaceuticals. Two radiopharmaceuticals are approved for pain palliation in patients with metastatic bone disease: ^{89}Sr-chloride (Metastron [GE Healthcare]) and ^{153}Sm-lexidronam (Quadramet [Berlex]). The benefits of radiopharmaceuticals for pain palliation include single-dose administration with up to 3 months of clinical effect, and systemic therapy that allows coverage of lesions throughout the body. Although the pain relief may not be complete, it should enable patients to reduce their dependence on narcotics and improve their overall quality of life. These radiopharmaceuticals cannot cure the disease but can decrease the pain associated with metastatic lesions in the bone.

Non-Hodgkin's Lymphoma

Non-Hodgkin's lymphoma (NHL) is the most common cancer affecting the blood and lymphatic system. Several treatment options are available, including radioimmunotherapy. ^{90}Y-radiolabeled ibritumomab tiuxetan (Zevalin [Cell Therapeutics and Spectrum Pharmaceuticals]) is indicated for relapsed or refractory, low-grade, follicular, or transformed B-cell NHL and rituximab-refractory follicular NHL. ^{131}I-radiolabeled tositumomab (Bexxar [Corixa and GlaxoSmithKline]) is indicated for patients who have CD20-positive follicular NHL with or without transformation and whose disease is refractory to rituximab and relapsed after chemotherapy. Like the nonradioactive immunotherapy agent rituximab, the monoclonal antibody nature of both of these radiopharmaceuticals allows for targeted therapy at the site of the disease. In general, immunotherapy agents work by enhancing and supplementing the body's own immune response in fighting off disease. However, in many patients, immunotherapy stops being effective at some point. The radioactive therapy agents for NHL share the monoclonal antibody component, which stimulates the body's immune response, and both of these radiopharmaceuticals are labeled with fairly high-energy beta-emitting isotopes that kill off tumor cells as a result of the beta emissions. Both ^{131}I and ^{90}Y emit beta particles that will penetrate several cell widths, allowing delivery of therapeutic levels of radiation to cells that are in the center of the tumor mass and may not completely benefit from the immunotherapy portion of the treatment.

Isotope Shortage

In recent years, the nuclear medicine community has experienced the most severe isotope shortages in history. In May 2009 the Canadian National Research Universal (NRU) reactor in Chalk River, Ontario, was shut down because of a pinhole-size water leak. The NRU reactor supplied the world with one-third of its radioisotopes for nuclear imaging studies. The shortage was compounded by the shutdown of the Dutch High Flux Reactor in Petten, which supplies the world with another one-third of its medical isotopes. This left the smaller Belgian, French, and South African reactors to try to meet the needs of the entire nuclear medicine community. The result was severe shortages of the most common radioisotope, ^{99m}Tc. For more than a year, clinicians and nuclear pharmacists were forced to struggle with a limited supply of radioactive materials to meet patient needs. All of the reactors came back on line in the second half of 2010, but this shortage has highlighted the fragile supply of this important isotope.

During the shortage, clinicians were forced to either order different diagnostic tests or postpone testing to work around isotope availability. Although the impact of this is not yet known, it is possible that some studies that had been routinely performed using nuclear medicine procedures are now being done with other imaging technologies. A benefit of the shortage was that in some cases, the lack of ^{99m}Tc led to an increase in the use of PET imaging for certain diseases. Regardless, maintaining an adequate supply of radioactive materials to prevent disruption of nuclear medicine imaging will continue to be of concern.

Conclusion

Despite the recent issues with supply, nuclear medicine as a diagnostic imaging modality continues to contribute greatly to the care of patients with a wide variety of diseases. The ability to image both anatomy and functional capacity of different organs and organ systems makes nuclear medicine a unique diagnostic option. The continuing migration toward PET will solidify the utility of this imaging modality and support its future use.

References

1. United States Nuclear Regulatory Commission. Biological effects of radiation. www.nrc.gov/reading-rm/doc-collections/fact-sheets/bio-effects-radiation.pdf. Accessed August 2011.
2. Kowalsky RJ, Falen SW, eds. *Radiopharmaceuticals in Nuclear Pharmacy and Nuclear Medicine.* 2nd ed. Washington, DC: American Pharmacists Association; 2004.
3. Brookhaven National Laboratory. The technetium-99m generator. www.bnl.gov/bnlweb/history/Tc-99m.asp. Accessed August 2010.
4. Early PJ, Sodee BD. *Principles and Practice of Nuclear Medicine.* St Louis: Mosby; 1995.
5. Pharmaceutical compounding—sterile preparations (general chapter 797). *The United States Pharmacopeia and The National Formulary.* Rockville, MD: United States Pharmacopeial Convention, Inc; 2004.
6. Tapscott E. Nuclear medicine pioneer, Hal O. Anger, 1920–2005. *J Nucl Med Technol.* 2005;33:250–3.
7. Ziessman HA. *Nuclear Medicine.* Philadelphia: Mosby; 2006.
8. Smith BT, ed. *Nuclear Pharmacy.* Gurnee, IL: Pharmaceutical Press; 2010.

CHAPTER 6

Radiopharmaceuticals Used in Nuclear Medicine Imaging

Wendy Galbraith and Allegra L. DePietro

Nuclear medicine is a medical specialty that uses very small amounts of radioactive materials (radiopharmaceuticals) along with imaging procedures to diagnose, manage, and treat disease. A radiopharmaceutical is a drug containing a radionuclide that is used in the nuclear medicine procedure for either diagnosis or treatment. Nuclear medicine or molecular imaging is a valuable modality used to gather medical information that otherwise would be unavailable, would require surgery, or would necessitate more expensive diagnostic tests. The use of radioactive material in medicine dates back to 1901, when radium was used to treat skin lesions.[1] Today nearly all hospitals, as well as many clinics and private physicians' offices, perform nuclear medicine tests and scans.

About 80% of nuclear medicine procedures use a radiopharmaceutical labeled with the radionuclide technetium 99m (^{99m}Tc). ^{99m}Tc is obtained from a generator system and then compounded with a chemical substance that, when administered, will have some affinity for an organ or tissue. Because ^{99m}Tc has a half-life of 6 hours, the radiopharmaceuticals labeled with this radionuclide must be compounded on the day of use.

The most notable use of radiopharmaceuticals for therapy is the treatment of thyroid disease with iodine 131 (^{131}I). Therapeutic radiopharmaceuticals used in the nuclear medicine department are termed "unsealed radioactive sources" and are administered intravenously or orally to the patient. The therapeutic use of radiopharmaceuticals is often confused with the external radiation treatments associated with radiation oncology.

Just as with medication therapy, it is important to select the correct imaging procedure and associated radiopharmaceutical to avoid unnecessary radiation exposure of the patient or delay in diagnosis and treatment. This chapter is intended to help practitioners recognize the influence of drugs and other factors that affect radiopharmaceutical administration, with the goal of increasing the diagnostic reliability of nuclear medicine procedures and providing guidance on differentiating true patient conditions. The chapter is organized into two sections. The first covers radiopharmaceuticals used for diagnosis; the drugs are listed alphabetically, starting with ^{99m}Tc-labeled radiopharmaceuticals and followed by radiopharmaceuticals labeled with other radionuclides. The second section covers radiopharmaceuticals used for therapy.

Radiopharmaceuticals Used for Diagnosis

Technetium Tc 99m Bicisate

Technetium Tc 99m bicisate (^{99m}Tc-bicisate, ^{99m}Tc-ECD, or ^{99m}Tc-ethyl cysteinate dimer; Neurolite [Lantheus]) is used as a diagnostic aid in cerebral vascular disease. It is indicated as an adjunct to magnetic resonance imaging (MRI) and computed tomography (CT) in the evaluation and localization of stroke and cerebral functional impairment including dementia, head trauma, and epilepsy.[2] It is also used in the clinical diagnosis of brain death.[1]

Dosage and Administration

The adult dosage for cerebral perfusion is 25 mCi via intravenous bolus, with a range of 10–30 mCi. The pediatric dosage is 0.2–0.3 mCi/kg, with a minimum dose of 3 mCi.[3]

For brain death, imaging takes place as the drug is being injected, followed by delayed images. For epilepsy, the drug must be injected within 30–60 seconds after the onset of the seizure, and imaging takes place 2–24 hours later. For all other indications, imaging takes place approximately 2 hours after injection.[4]

^{99m}Tc-bicisate has rapid blood clearance because of its lipophilic structure, and at 5 minutes after injection about 5%–7% of the administered activity localizes in the brain by passive diffusion.[5] At 1 hour after injection, normal biodistribution can be seen in the facial muscles, salivary glands, and blood pool (not protein bound). ^{99m}Tc-bicisate is eliminated primarily by the kidneys, with 50% eliminated in the first 2 hours. Some bowel elimination occurs, with about 12% excreted in 48 hours.[1]

Adverse Effects

Adverse effects, observed in less than 1% of patients, include angina, cardiac failure, apnea, headache, nausea, syncope, seizures, and rash.[6] The product kit contains the chelate EDTA; inconsistent changes in serum calcium and phosphate levels have been seen in fewer than 2% of patients.[2]

Contraindications

The only contraindication to ^{99m}Tc-bicisate injection is hypersensitivity to any agent in the kit.

Medication Therapy Management (MTM) Concerns

The FDA pregnancy category is C. Technetium, as free pertechnetate, crosses the placenta and is distributed into breast milk. The manufacturer recommends that breast-feeding be discontinued for 3 days.[2] No major drug interactions with ^{99m}Tc-bicisate have been reported. Acetazolamide may be used as an interventional agent to evaluate cerebral hemodynamic reserve. Patients should be well hydrated and should be encouraged to drink fluids and void frequently for 2–6 hours after administration.[4]

Technetium Tc 99m Disofenin

Technetium Tc 99m disofenin (^{99m}Tc-disofenin or ^{99m}Tc-DISIDA; Hepatolite [Pharmalucence]) is used in the evaluation of hepatobiliary disorders, including tract patency and bile leaks. It can be used in pediatric patients to differentiate between biliary atresia and neonatal hepatitis, when combined with phenobarbital treatment.

Dosage and Administration

The adult dosage is 3–10 mCi administered intravenously. The pediatric dosage is 0.05–0.07 mCi/kg (dosage adjustments based on age or body surface area [BSA] may also be used), with a minimum activity of 0.5 mCi. A minimum activity of 1 mCi may be used when bilirubin is elevated.[7]

Imaging is performed immediately after administration of the radiopharmaceutical and is usually completed in 60–90 minutes. Imaging up to 4 hours or longer may be necessary if no activity is seen in the gallbladder or intestines. After activity is seen in the gallbladder and intestines, the patient is given an interventional agent, sincalide, to stimulate gallbladder contraction. The patient is again imaged for approximately 30 minutes to determine the gallbladder ejection fraction.[8]

Within 10 minutes after intravenous injection of ^{99m}Tc-disofenin, 80% of the injected dose is taken up in the liver, with about 8% remaining in circulation at 30 minutes.[9] Elimination is predominantly by the bowel, with about 9% elimination by the kidneys within 2 hours after injection.[10]

Adverse Effects

Adverse effects are rare but include chills, nausea and vomiting, erythema multiforme, and pain at the injection site.[10]

Contraindications

The only contraindication to a ^{99m}Tc-disofenin injection is hypersensitivity to any agent in the kit.

MTM Concerns

The FDA pregnancy category is C. Technetium, as free pertechnetate, crosses the placenta and is distributed into breast milk.[10] Breast-feeding should be interrupted for 4 hours.[11] The patient should fast for at least 2–5 hours but not longer than 12 hours. Also, patients should not be taking pain medications that contain opium or morphine derivatives for 2–6 hours before the study.[8] Pediatric patients must be treated with 5 mg/kg/day of phenobarbital for 3–5 days prior to the imaging procedure to differentiate between biliary atresia and neonatal hepatitis.[12] Drug interactions with ^{99m}Tc-disofenin have been reported. Opioid (narcotic) analgesics, especially meperidine or morphine derivatives, will delay intestinal transit of the imaging agent and may result in nonvisualization of the bowel. Hepatic artery infusion of chemotherapy and total parenteral nutrition result in absent or delayed visualization of the gallbladder in patients with no gallbladder disease. Somatostatin, anticholinergics, erythromycin, and high doses of nicotinic acid will interfere with the study.[9]

Technetium Tc 99m Exametazime

Technetium Tc 99m exametazime (^{99m}Tc-exametazime, ^{99m}Tc-HMPAO, or ^{99m}Tc-hexamethylpropyleneamine oxime; Ceretec [GE Healthcare]) is indicated as an adjunct to MRI and CT in evaluation and localization of stroke and cerebral functional impairment including dementia, head trauma, and epilepsy. It is also used in the clinical diagnosis of brain death.[1] Unstabilized ^{99m}Tc-exametazime is indicated for the labeling of white blood cells (WBCs) for localization of inflammation.[13]

Dosage and Administration

The dosage for cerebral perfusion is 10–30 mCi of stabilized ^{99m}Tc-exametazime administered intravenously through a 0.45-µm filter. The dosage of ^{99m}Tc-exametazime-labeled WBCs is 10–20 mCi.[13] The pediatric dosage for cerebral perfusion is 0.2–0.3 mCi/kg, with a minimum dose of 3 mCi. The pediatric dosage for labeled WBCs is 0.1–0.2 mCi/kg, with a minimum dose of 0.5 mCi.[3,14]

For brain death, imaging takes place as the drug is being injected, followed by delayed images. For epilepsy, the drug must be injected within 30–60 seconds after the onset of the seizure, and the imaging takes place 2–24 hours later. For all other indications, imaging is performed approximately 2 hours after injection.[4] For infection imaging, approximately 60 mL of blood must be withdrawn from the patient for radiolabeling. Isolation of the WBCs, labeling time, and transportation to a nuclear pharmacy, if used, result in a 2–3 hour delay before the labeled radiopharmaceutical is ready for injection into the patient. Imaging can begin 1–2 hours after injection.[8]

^{99m}Tc-exametazime is injected intravenously and has rapid blood clearance, with about 3.5%–7% of the activity localizing in the brain by passive diffusion in 5 minutes.[5] ^{99m}Tc-exametazime is retained in the brain tissue because of intracellular conversion by glutathione oxidation to a hydrophilic compound that diffuses poorly across cell membranes. ^{99m}Tc-exametazime is eliminated about half through the kidneys and half through the bowel by 48 hours.[1] The lipophilic ^{99m}Tc-exametazime complex (which is not stabilized by methylene blue) is taken up by leukocytes and selectively retained in neutrophils. During the first hour after intravenous administration of ^{99m}Tc-exametazime-labeled WBCs, activity is seen in the lungs, liver, spleen, blood pool, bone marrow, and bladder.[13] Bowel activity is routinely visualized by 3–4 hours and increases with time.[5] For labeled leukocytes, about 15%–30% of the administered activity is excreted renally in 24 hours and about 6% is eliminated via the bowel in 48 hours.[9]

Adverse Effects

Reported adverse effects include an 8% frequency of transient increase in blood pressure and less than 1% frequency of rash, facial edema, and fever.[13] Other reported adverse effects include anaphylaxis, hypotension, seizures, facial swelling, abdominal pain, and dyspnea with myoclonus (labeled WBCs).[6]

Contraindications

The only contraindication to ^{99m}Tc-exametazime injection is hypersensitivity to any agent in the kit.

MTM Concerns

The FDA pregnancy category is C. Technetium, as free pertechnetate, crosses the placenta and is distributed into breast milk. The manufacturer recommends that breast-feeding be discontinued for 2.5 days after the study.[13] Patients should be well hydrated and should be encouraged to drink fluids and void frequently for 2–6 hours after administration.[4] No major drug interactions have been reported with ^{99m}Tc-exametazime for cerebral studies. Acetazolamide may be used as an interventional agent to evaluate cerebral hemodynamic reserve. With labeled leukocytes, several drugs can have an effect on the biodistribution of the leukocytes in vivo, and a few drugs can affect the labeling efficiency of ^{99m}Tc-exametazime to WBCs. Antibiotics, corticosteroids, total parenteral nutrition, lidocaine, procainamide, epinephrine, interferon, interleukin, and radiation therapy have been found to affect labeled leukocyte biodistribution.[15,16] Drugs shown to decrease labeling efficiency include acetaminophen and acid citrate dextrose.[15]

Technetium Tc 99m Macroaggregated Albumin (MAA)

Technetium Tc 99m-labeled macroaggregated albumin particles, or ^{99m}Tc-MAA, are used in lung perfusion imaging, LeVeen (peritoneal) shunt assessment, venogram scintigraphy, and right-to-left cardiac shunt assessment.[17]

Dosage and Administration

The ^{99m}Tc-MAA dosage is dependent on activity and number of particles. In adults without pulmonary hypertension, the dosage is 3–5 mCi if administered postventilation and 1–3 mCi if administered preventilation. The particle count for an adult should be between 150,000 and 500,000[18] (200,000–700,000 in the Pulmolite [Pharmlucence] package insert). The number of particles must be decreased to 100,000 in patients with right-to-left shunt. In pediatric patients, the particle count and dosage should be decreased, for example, to a minimum activity of 0.3 mCi and 10,000–50,000 particles for patients less than 1 year of age.[17]

Lung perfusion using ^{99m}Tc-MAA is usually accompanied by a ventilation procedure using either radioactive xenon 133 (^{133}Xe) gas or aerosolized ^{99m}Tc-pentetate (DTPA) administered via inhalation, with the ventilation procedure performed before administration of ^{99m}Tc-MAA. Images are obtained immediately after intravenous administration of ^{99m}Tc-MAA, with the patient supine, over 10–15 minutes. No special patient preparation is necessary.

Immediately after injection, 80% of the administered activity is retained in the pulmonary alveolar capillary bed by physical blockade. The particles undergo erosion and fragmentation to the reticuloendothelial system in 30 minutes, with an effective half-life of 3 hours. Greater than 75% of the ^{99m}Tc portion is eliminated via the kidneys in the first 24 hours.[17]

Adverse Effects

Rare instances of hemodynamic and idiosyncratic reactions to ^{99m}Tc-MAA have occurred.[8] Adverse effects also include cardiac arrest, chest pain, hypertension, hypotension, tachycardia, anaphylaxis, cyanosis, flushing, chills, nausea, metallic taste, dyspnea, and diffuse rash.[6]

Contraindications

^{99m}Tc-MAA is contraindicated in patients with hypersensitivity to human serum albumin and those with severe pulmonary hypertension.[17]

MTM Concerns

The FDA pregnancy category is C. Technetium, as free pertechnetate, crosses the placenta and is distributed into breast milk. Breast-feeding should be discontinued for 12 hours after administration.[11] A particle count between 60,000 and 125,000 should be used in patients with right-to-left cardiac shunt.[9] A drug interaction with heparin results in the appearance of a perfusion image typically observed with pulmonary emboli.[16] Interactions with albumin, magnesium sulfate in pediatric patients, and methotrexate have also been reported.[15]

Technetium Tc 99m Mebrofenin

Technetium Tc 99m mebrofenin (^{99m}Tc-mebrofenin or ^{99m}Tc-BROMIDA; Choletec [Bracco]) is used in the evaluation of hepatobiliary disorders, including tract patency and bile leaks. It can be used in pediatric patients to differentiate between biliary atresia and neonatal hepatitis when combined with phenobarbital treatment.

Dosage and Administration

The adult dosage is 3–10 mCi administered intravenously. The pediatric dosage is 0.05–0.07 mCi/kg (age-based or BSA-based adjustments may also be used), with a minimum activity of 0.5 mCi. A minimum activity of 1 mCi may be used if bilirubin is elevated.[7]

Imaging is performed immediately after administration of the radiopharmaceutical and is usually completed in 60–90 minutes. Imaging up to 4 hours or longer may be necessary if no activity is seen in the gallbladder or intestines. After activity is seen in the gallbladder and intestines, the patient is given an interventional agent, sincalide, to stimulate gallbladder contraction. The patient is again imaged for approximately 30 minutes to determine the gallbladder ejection fraction.[8]

Immediately after injection, 80% of the dosage is seen in the hepatobiliary system via liver accumulation within 10 minutes, and 17% remains in circulation. This tracer has less competitive binding for bilirubin than the other hepatobiliary tracer, disofenin. With increasing bilirubin levels, the tracer will increasingly be excreted via the kidneys. Normal biodistribution is seen in the blood, kidneys, and hepatobiliary system. Elimination is predominantly via the bowel, with about 1% elimination via the kidneys in 3 hours after injection.[19]

Adverse Effects

Adverse effects are rare, but urticaria/hives has been reported.[6]

Contraindications

The only contraindication to ^{99m}Tc-mebrofenin injection is hypersensitivity to any agent in the kit.

MTM Concerns

The FDA pregnancy category is C. Technetium, as free pertechnetate, crosses the placenta and is distributed into breast milk.[19] Breast-feeding should be interrupted for 4 hours.[11] The patient should fast for at least 2–5 hours but not longer than 12 hours. Also, patients should not be taking pain medications that contain opium or morphine derivatives for 2–6 hours before the study.[8] Pediatric patients must be treated with 5 mg/kg/day of phenobarbital for 3–5 days prior to the imaging procedure to differentiate between biliary atresia and neonatal hepatitis.[12] Drug interactions have been reported with ^{99m}Tc-mebrofenin. Opioid (narcotic) analgesics, especially meperidine or morphine derivatives, will delay intestinal transit of the imaging agent and may result in nonvisualization of the bowel. Hepatic artery infusion of chemotherapy and total parenteral nutrition result in absent or delayed visualization of the gallbladder in patients with no gallbladder disease. Somatostatin, anticholinergics, erythromycin, and high doses of nicotinic acid will interfere with the study.[9]

Technetium Tc 99m Medronate

Technetium Tc 99m medronate (^{99m}Tc-medronate or ^{99m}Tc-MDP) is used in the diagnosis of bone disease, including metastatic lesions, and determination of osteomyelitis.

Dosage and Administration

The adult dosage for skeletal imaging is 15–30 mCi. The pediatric dosage is 200 µCi × weight in kilograms or 20 mCi × BSA/1.73 m^2, with a minimum activity of 3 mCi.[20]

For dynamic flow studies, imaging takes place during ^{99m}Tc-MDP administration. For blood pool data, images are taken statically for 15 minutes. In most cases imaging will begin 2–3 hours after administration and last for 20–30 minutes.

^{99m}Tc-MDP is administered intravenously, and skeletal uptake occurs as a function of blood flow to bone and ion exchange during osteoblastic activity. The diphosphonate compound is exchanged for calcium in the formation of hydroxyapatite crystals.[9] By 3 hours postadministration approximately 50% of the activity is excreted via the kidneys and approximately 50% is seen in the skeleton. Soft-tissue uptake can increase with decreased renal function or dehydration.[21]

Adverse Effects

Adverse effects are rare but include cardiac arrest, chest pain, tachycardia, seizures, hypotension, hypertension, dizziness, flushing, diffuse rash, urticaria, chills, nausea and vomiting, headache, metallic taste, and asthenia.[6,21]

Contraindications

The only contraindication to ^{99m}Tc-MDP injection is hypersensitivity to any agent in the kit.

MTM Concerns

The FDA pregnancy category is C. Technetium, as free pertechnetate, crosses the placenta and is distributed into breast milk.[21] Breast-feeding should be interrupted for 4 hours.[11] Except that the patient be well hydrated, no special preparation is needed. After administration patients should be instructed to drink fluids and void frequently for 2–6 hours. Caution should be used in patients with possible or diagnosed hypocalcemia.[21] Drug interactions have been reported with iron-containing compounds, potassium and sodium phosphates, corticosteroids, and nifedipine.[22] Interactions with the acute administration of bisphosphonates vary; etidronate decreases sensitivity while alendronate and zoledronic acid do not appear to alter bone scan results.[23] Interactions have also been reported with amphotericin B, gentamicin, cyclophosphamide, vincristine, and doxorubicin; these drugs can increase renal retention of the radiopharmaceutical.[16] Aluminum-containing antacids and sodium diatrizoate will increase liver accumulation.[9]

Technetium Tc 99m Mertiatide

Technetium Tc 99m mertiatide (^{99m}Tc-mertiatide, ^{99m}Tc-mercaptoacetyltriglycine, or ^{99m}Tc-MAG3) is used for evaluation of renal function, including effective renal plasma flow, urinary tract obstruction, and split kidney function,[24] and for diagnosis of renovascular hypertension.[25]

Dosage and Administration

The adult dosage is 5–10 mCi and the pediatric dosage is 50–100 μCi/kg with a minimum dosage of 1 mCi and a maximum activity of 5 mCi.[26]

Imaging is started while ^{99m}Tc-MAG3 is injected intravenously and continues for 1 hour. Frequently, a diuretic may be administered halfway into the study to differentiate dilation of the renal collecting system from obstruction.[8] An angiotensin-converting enzyme (ACE) inhibitor (captopril or enalapril) is used in conjunction with ^{99m}Tc-MAG3 to diagnose renovascular hypertension.

^{99m}Tc-mertiatide is highly protein bound, which is reversible, and 98% of the injected activity undergoes tubular secretion with no reabsorption, while 2% is excreted through glomerular filtration. Ninety percent of the injected activity is excreted within 3 hours. With decreasing renal function, hepatobiliary excretion will increase.[24]

Adverse Effects

Adverse effects are rare but include nausea, vomiting, wheezing, dyspnea, itching, rash, flushing, tachycardia, hypertension, shaking, chills, fever, and seizures.[24]

Contraindications

The only contraindication to ^{99m}Tc-mertiatide injection is hypersensitivity to any agent in the kit.[24]

MTM Concerns

The FDA pregnancy category is C. Technetium, as free pertechnetate, crosses the placenta and is distributed into breast milk.[24] Breast-feeding should be interrupted for 24 hours.[9] Patients should be well hydrated and should be asked to empty their bladder prior to beginning the study. Patients may or may not be asked to stay off their medications, depending on the physician's preference. No major drug interactions have been reported with ^{99m}Tc-mertiatide. Drugs that have effects on the renal system will alter the distribution of the radiotracer; these include iodinated contrast agents, aminoglycosides, cyclosporine, cisplatin, furosemide, ACE inhibitors, and probenecid. ACE inhibitors and angiotensin II blockers should be stopped before imaging for renovascular hypertension.

Technetium Tc 99m Oxidronate

Technetium Tc 99m oxidronate (^{99m}Tc-oxidronate or ^{99m}Tc-HDP) is used in the diagnosis of bone disease, including metastatic lesions, and determination of osteomyelitis.

Dosage and Administration

The adult dosage for skeletal imaging is 15–30 mCi. The pediatric dosage is 200 μCi × weight in kilograms or 20 mCi × BSA/1.73 m^2, with a minimum activity of 3 mCi.[20]

For dynamic flow studies, imaging takes place during ^{99m}Tc-HDP administration. For blood pool data, images are taken statically for 15 minutes. In most cases imaging will begin 2–3 hours after administration and last for 20–30 minutes.

^{99m}Tc-HDP is administered intravenously, and skeletal system uptake occurs as a function of blood flow to bone and ion exchange during osteoblastic activity. The diphosphonate compound is exchanged for calcium in the formation of hydroxyapatite crystals. By 2 hours postadministration approximately 50% of the activity is excreted via the kidneys and approximately 50% is seen in the skeleton. Soft-tissue uptake can increase with decreased renal function or dehydration.[27]

Adverse Effects

Adverse effects are rare but include nausea; vomiting; erythema; flushing; diffuse rash; pruritus; chest pain, tightness, or heaviness; heartburn; seizures; diaphoresis; and facial swelling.[6]

Contraindications

The only contraindication to ^{99m}Tc-HDP injection is hypersensitivity to any agent in the kit.

MTM Concerns

The FDA pregnancy category is C. Technetium, as free pertechnetate, crosses the placenta and is distributed into breast milk.[27] Breast-feeding should be interrupted for 4 hours.[11] Except that the patient be well hydrated, no special preparation is needed. After administration, patients should be instructed to drink fluids and to void frequently for 2–6 hours. Caution should be used in patients with possible or diagnosed hypocalcemia. Drug interactions have been reported with iron-containing compounds, potassium and sodium phosphates, corticosteroids, and nifedipine.[22] Interactions with the acute administration of bisphosphonates vary; etidronate decreases sensitivity, while alendronate and zoledronic acid do not appear to alter bone scan results.[23] Interactions have also been reported with amphotericin B, gentamicin, cyclophosphamide, vincristine, and doxorubicin; these drugs can increase renal retention of the radiopharmaceutical.[16] Aluminum-containing antacids and sodium diatrizoate will increase liver accumulation.[9]

Technetium Tc 99m Pentetate

Technetium Tc 99m pentetate (^{99m}Tc-pentetate or ^{99m}Tc-DTPA) is used to evaluate renal function, including glomerular filtration, urinary tract obstruction, and split kidney function. ^{99m}Tc-DTPA is also used for lung ventilation studies when aerosolized, for cardiac first-pass studies to determine right and left ventricular ejection fraction, and as a conventional brain imaging agent.

Dosage and Administration

The adult dosage for renal imaging is 5–10 mCi administered intravenously (pediatric renal dosage is 100–200 μCi/kg with a minimum of 1 mCi). The adult dosage for pulmonary disease is 30–50 mCi aerosolized for inhalation. The adult dosage for cardiac first-pass studies is 15–25 mCi administered by intravenous bolus.

For renal and first-pass cardiac studies, imaging is started while ^{99m}Tc-DTPA is injected intravenously. Frequently, a diuretic may be administered halfway into the study to differentiate dilation of the renal collecting system from obstruction.[8]

After intravenous injection, ^{99m}Tc-DTPA is cleared from circulation within the first 5 minutes and undergoes 100% glomerular filtration. Ninety percent of the injected activity is excreted within 4 hours, with a biologic half-life of 2.5 hours.[28]

Adverse Effects

Adverse effects are rare but include chills, nausea, and urticaria at injection.[28]

Contraindications

The only contraindication to ^{99m}Tc-DTPA injection is hypersensitivity to any agent in the kit.

MTM Concerns

The FDA pregnancy category is C. Technetium, as free pertechnetate, crosses the placenta and is distributed into breast milk.[28] Breast-feeding should be interrupted for 12 hours.[11] Patients should be well hydrated and should be asked to empty their bladder prior to beginning the study. Patients may or may not be asked to stay off their medications, depending on the physician's preference. Interactions have been reported with aluminum-containing drugs, nephrotoxic drugs, dipyridamole, and ACE inhibitors.[22] ACE inhibitors may be used as interventional agents in renal scintigraphy.

Technetium Tc 99m Sodium Pertechnetate

Sodium pertechnetate Tc 99m (^{99m}Tc-sodium pertechnetate, $Na^{99m}TcO_4$, "tech," or "free tech") is used for various imaging studies and as the starting material for labeling many of the diagnostic agents used in nuclear medicine.

Dosage and Administration

Adult dosages for various studies are as follows: thyroid studies, 2–10 mCi intravenously; blood pool studies as labeled red blood cells (RBCs), 10–30 mCi intravenously; direct cystography, 1 mCi instilled through a bladder catheter; evaluation of the salivary system, 1 mCi administered orally; brain imaging, 20–30 mCi intravenously; and dacryoscintigraphy imaging, 100 µCi/drop applied in each eye.[29] Pediatric dosages use a fraction of the adult activity, based on the child's BSA or weight, with a minimum amount of activity required for neonates.[29]

The most common types of studies using pertechnetate are thyroid imaging, cardiac function or gastric bleeding studies using labeled RBCs (see Technetium Tc 99m Red Blood Cells), and cystography in children. Thyroid imaging begins approximately 30 minutes after intravenous administration of ^{99m}Tc-sodium pertechnetate and lasts for approximately 30 minutes. For cystography, the patient is catheterized and a saline intravenous solution is used to fill the bladder via the catheter. The radiopharmaceutical is diluted in the saline. Study time can vary and depends on endpoints for the patient.[8]

When injected intravenously or taken orally, ^{99m}Tc-sodium pertechnetate accumulates in the thyroid (trapped and released unchanged), salivary glands, choroid plexus, gastric mucosa, intracranial lesions, and blood pool and is excreted by the kidneys.[29]

Adverse Effects

Allergic reactions, including anaphylaxis, have occurred.[29] Other reported side effects are chills; nausea; vomiting; diffuse rash; pruritus; hives/urticaria; chest pain, tightness, or heaviness; hypertension; dizziness; vertigo; headache; and diaphoresis.[6]

Contraindications

The only contraindication to ^{99m}Tc-sodium pertechnetate injection is hypersensitivity to a previous sodium pertechnetate injection.[29]

MTM Concerns

The FDA pregnancy category is C. Technetium, as free pertechnetate, crosses the placenta and is distributed into breast milk.[29] Breast-feeding should be interrupted for 24 hours for intravenous pertechnetate studies.[11] For thyroid evaluation, patient preparation is critical. Medications given to patients with thyroid conditions, along with some vitamins, foods, and iodinated contrast media, may alter radiopharmaceutical uptake. Altered uptake in thyroid studies has been reported with antithyroid drugs (propylthiouracil), iodine-containing compounds (Lugol's solution and vitamin preparations), iodine ointment, antitussives, amiodarone, iodinated contrast media, thyroid supplements, meprobamate, phenylbutazone, corticosteroids, adrenocorticotrophic hormone, sulfonamides, perchlorate, and antihistamines.[22] Interactions have been reported with aluminum-containing antacids, stannous ion-containing drugs, and other radiopharmaceuticals, resulting in failure of the radiopharmaceutical to leave the vascular space and increased blood pool activity.[29]

Technetium Tc 99m Pyrophosphate

In the past, labeled pyrophosphate, as ^{99m}Tc-PYP (^{99m}Tc-PPi), was used in the evaluation of infarcted myocardial tissue and in skeletal imaging. ^{99m}Tc-PYP is no longer used for these indications. The unlabeled pyrophosphate (PYP) kit is used mostly for its stannous-ion content for labeling RBCs for blood pool imaging, including resting nuclear ventriculography (RNVG), and to a lesser extent for imaging gastrointestinal (GI) bleeding and hemangiomas. (See Technetium Tc 99m Red Blood Cells.)

Technetium Tc 99m Red Blood Cells

Technetium Tc 99m-labeled RBCs (^{99m}Tc-RBCs) are used for blood pool imaging. Blood pool agents are used in assessment of myocardial wall motion abnormalities, measurement of ventricular ejection fraction, and volume in RNVG studies. Blood pool agents are also frequently used in the assessment of GI bleeding. RNVG studies are the principal application of the in vivo labeling method using the PYP kit. GI studies are the principal application of the in vitro method using the UltraTag kit (Covidien).

Dosage and Administration

The adult administered activity is usually 15–25 mCi. Administered activity in children should be reduced according to BSA or weight. The minimum pediatric administered activity should be as low as practically achievable for appropriate image quality.[30]

For localization of GI bleeding, the patient's RBCs are labeled and reinjected. The labeling process takes approximately 40 minutes and, after intravenous administration, the imaging may take 60 minutes depending on the endpoints.[8]

The PYP kit is used for RBC labeling with an in vivo method. In this process ^{99m}Tc diffuses across the RBC membrane and is reduced by the previously injected stannous ion, whereby it binds to hemoglobin; this prevents it from diffusing back out of the cell. Approximately 78% of the injected activity remains in the blood pool. The biologic half-life of ^{99m}Tc-RBCs is about 80 days with the in vivo method.[31]

With the in vitro (UltraTag) method, after intravenous injection the ^{99m}Tc-RBCs distribute in the blood pool with an estimated biologic half-life of 29 hours. Ninety-five percent of ^{99m}Tc remains bound to RBCs 24 hours after injection.[32]

Adverse Effects

Allergic reactions, skin rash, hives, and itching have been reported.[9]

Contraindications

The only contraindication to ^{99m}Tc-RBC injection is hypersensitivity to any agent in the kits.[32]

MTM Concerns

The FDA pregnancy category is C. Technetium, as free pertechnetate, crosses the placenta and is distributed into breast milk.[32] Breast-feeding should be interrupted for 12 hours for ^{99m}Tc-RBC studies.[11] The in vivo method cannot be used for GI bleeding because variable amounts of technetium localize in the gastric mucosa and interfere with imaging and because radioactivity is eliminated via the urinary tract. In vivo labeling of RBCs can be affected by many drugs and processes, including dipyridamole, recent administration of iodinated contrast agents, and dialysis. Antibodies directed against the RBC membrane in patients with chronic lymphocytic leukemia or non-Hodgkin's lymphoma may result in poor labeling. If a patient has received a recent blood transfusion, is in renal failure, or is on heparin or doxorubicin, the in vivo technique may result in unacceptably high levels of unbound technetium.[30] Poor labeling can result from administration of digoxin, hydralazine, methyldopa, nifedipine, quinidine, prazosin, or iodinated radiopaque agents as well as extreme deviations in amounts of stannous ion or sodium pertechnetate.[31] Beta-blockers, nitrates, and calcium antagonists when used for exercise nuclear ventriculography will mask disease.[22]

Technetium Tc 99m Sestamibi

Technetium Tc 99m sestamibi (^{99m}Tc-sestamibi or ^{99m}Tc-MIBI; Cardiolite and Miraluma [Lantheus]) is used in myocardial perfusion imaging to assess the severity and localization of myocardial infarction or myocardial ischemia, to determine left ventricular ejection fraction, to assess ventricular wall motion, and to assess coronary artery disease. ^{99m}Tc-sestamibi is also used to assess hyperparathyroidism. Miraluma is used in postmammography detection and localization of breast carcinoma.[33]

Dosage and Administration

The adult dosage for myocardial perfusion imaging involves the injection of two doses of ^{99m}Tc-sestamibi. If a 1-day protocol is used the adult doses are 8–15 mCi for the resting phase and three times the resting activity (24–45 mCi) for the exercise phase. The recommended total daily activity is 40 mCi. For parathyroid imaging the adult dose is 20–30 mCi, and for breast imaging the adult dose is up to 30 mCi. Administered activity in children should be reduced on the basis of weight or BSA and should be as low as practically achievable for appropriate image quality.[30]

A patient may undergo treadmill stress or chemical stress (using regadenoson, adenosine, dipyridamole, or dobutamine), depending on the patient's physiologic and mental state. To allow the tracer to clear from the liver and bowel, imaging takes place 15–45 minutes after intravenous administration of the dose and may take up to 30 minutes. The same procedure is followed for the resting phase of the study, which usually takes place prior to the exercise or stress phase.[30]

^{99m}Tc-sestamibi is injected intravenously and has a high volume of distribution. About 1.2% of the injected dose accumulates in the myocyte mitochondria. Normal biodistribution is to the hepatobiliary and cardiac systems, salivary glands, and thyroid. ^{99m}Tc-sestamibi is eliminated through the biliary system into the intestines. At 48 hours 27% of the injected activity is excreted by the kidneys and 33% by the bowel. The effective half-life is 3 hours in the myocardium and 28 minutes in the liver.[33]

Adverse Effects

The most frequent adverse effect is a metallic or bitter taste after injection. Adverse effects less frequently reported are flushing, headache and nausea, skin rash, angina, and ST segment changes.[33]

Contraindications

The only contraindication to ^{99m}Tc-sestamibi injection is hypersensitivity to any agent in the kit.

MTM Concerns

The FDA pregnancy category is C. Technetium, as free pertechnetate, crosses the placenta and is distributed into breast milk.[33] Breast-feeding should be interrupted for 4 hours for ^{99m}Tc-sestamibi studies.[11] Beta-blocking and calcium-channel-blocking medications often prevent the patient from achieving the desired heart rate and may reduce the sensitivity of the test. Depending on the clinical necessity or the clinical question, these agents may need to be discontinued by the patient's physician prior to examination for a time sufficient to obviate their pharmacologic effect. Patients should fast for at least 4 hours prior to exercise or pharmacologic stress.[30]

Technetium Tc 99m Succimer

Technetium Tc 99m succimer (^{99m}Tc-succimer or ^{99m}Tc-DMSA) is used in the evaluation of renal parenchymal disorders, including renal cortex scarring.

Dosage and Administration

The adult dosage is 5 mCi and the pediatric dosage is 0.05–0.1 mCi/kg, with a minimum of 0.3–1 mCi.[26]

Imaging is obtained 1–3 hours after ^{99m}Tc-DMSA intravenous injection. If there is significant hydronephrosis, delaying images 4–24 hours after injection or administering furosemide may be helpful.

^{99m}Tc-DMSA activity is cleared from the plasma with a half-time of about 60 minutes, and 50% of the injected activity concentrates in the renal cortex. Approximately 16% of the activity is excreted in the urine within 2 hours. At 6 hours about 20% of the dose is concentrated in each kidney.[34]

Adverse Effects

Adverse effects are rare and include syncope, abdominal pain, fever, nausea, and maculopapular skin rash.[6,34]

Contraindications

The only contraindication to ^{99m}Tc-DMSA injection is hypersensitivity to any agent in the kit.

MTM Concerns

There is no special patient preparation. Interactions with aluminum chloride and sodium bicarbonate, causing a decrease in renal distribution and an increase in hepatic distribution, have been reported. Captopril has caused decreased renal uptake.[22]

Technetium Tc 99m Sulfur Colloid

Technetium Tc 99m sulfur colloid (^{99m}Tc-sulfur colloid or ^{99m}Tc-SC) is used in the evaluation of several disorders. It is most frequently used for evaluation of lymph node involvement in metastatic disease. Its second most common use is evaluation of gastroesophageal disorders. It is used infrequently for evaluation of hepatic, splenic, and bone marrow diseases.

Dosage and Administration

Adult doses are as follows: liver/spleen (1–8 mCi intravenously), bone marrow (3–12 mCi intravenously), gastroesophageal motility (150–300 μCi orally), pulmonary aspiration (300–500 μCi orally), LeVeen shunts (1–3 mCi intraperitoneally), lymphoscintigraphy (0.4–1 mCi by subcutaneous injection), and profuse GI bleeding (10 mCi intravenously).

For lymphoscintigraphy, a preparation of filtered or unfiltered ^{99m}Tc-SC is administered in up to four injections around the lesion of interest. The administration technique is dependent on the type of malignancy and the physician's preference. The study is performed to locate the first draining lymph node(s) for easier localization and removal during surgery. Imaging may be performed 15 minutes after administration of the radiopharmaceutical. When the radiopharmaceutical has been allowed to migrate, the patient is taken to the surgical suite and the surgeon locates the sentinel node with an intraoperative probe. There is no special patient preparation for this procedure.[8]

When ^{99m}Tc-SC is administered orally, either as a liquid or as a solid incorporated into a meal, imaging can take place immediately. Patients are asked not to eat or drink for 6–8 hours and may be asked to stop taking any drugs affecting gastric motility. The patient ingests a ^{99m}Tc-SC-labeled meal (chicken liver, eggs, or oatmeal) over 10–15 minutes so imaging can begin before gastric emptying takes place. The patient is imaged for approximately 90 minutes.[8]

Intravenously administered ^{99m}Tc-SC is selectively concentrated in the reticuloendothelial system by phagocytic cells of the liver (80%–90% of injected dose), spleen (5%–10%), and bone marrow (1%–10%) within 15 minutes.[35]

Adverse Effects

Adverse effects include cardiopulmonary arrest, seizures, anaphylaxis, hypertension, hypotension, tachycardia, dyspnea, abdominal pain, fever, chills, bronchospasm, nausea, vomiting, perspiration, headache, redness, urticaria, numbness, dizziness, and burning at the injection site.[6,35]

Contraindications

The only contraindication to ^{99m}Tc-SC injection is hypersensitivity to any agent in the kit.

MTM Concerns

The FDA pregnancy category is C. Technetium, as free pertechnetate, crosses the placenta and is distributed into breast milk.[35] Breast-feeding should be interrupted for 4 hours when ^{99m}Tc-SC is administered intravenously.[11] With ^{99m}Tc-SC administered intravenously, drug interactions have caused decreased distribution to the liver, shifting to the spleen and bone marrow, and, in one case, pulmonary accumulation. These interactions involved antacids (aluminum and magnesium salts), methotrexate, carmustine, lomustine, anesthetic agents (halothane), estrogens, and androgens.[22] Drugs that can affect gastric emptying studies include atropine, propantheline, levodopa, albuterol, isoproterenol, narcotic analgesics, total parenteral nutrition, chlordiazepoxide–clidinium (Librax), glucose, antacids, cimetidine, erythromycin, histamine, metoclopramide, nifedipine, propranolol, and sucralfate.[15]

Technetium Tc 99m Tetrofosmin

Technetium Tc 99m tetrofosmin (^{99m}Tc-tetrofosmin; Myoview [GE Healthcare]) is used in myocardial perfusion imaging to assess the severity and localization of myocardial infarction and myocardial ischemia, to determine left ventricular ejection fraction, to assess ventricular wall motion, and to assess coronary artery disease.

Dosage and Administration

The adult dosage for myocardial perfusion imaging involves the injection of two doses of ^{99m}Tc-tetrofosmin. If a 1-day protocol is used the adult doses are 8–15 mCi for the resting phase and three times the resting activity (24–45 mCi) for the exercise phase. The recommended total daily activity is 40 mCi. Administered activity in children should be reduced on the basis of weight or BSA and should be as low as practically achievable for appropriate image quality.[30]

A patient may undergo treadmill stress or chemical stress (using regadenoson, adenosine, dipyridamole, or dobutamine), depending on the patient's physiologic and mental state. To allow the tracer to clear from the liver and bowel, imaging takes place 15–45 minutes after intravenous administration of the dose and may take up to 30 minutes. The same procedure is followed for the resting phase of the study, which usually takes place prior to the exercise or stress phase.[30]

^{99m}Tc-tetrofosmin is injected intravenously and has a high volume of distribution. About 1.2% of the injected dose accumulates in the myocyte cytoplasm. Normal biodistribution is to the hepatobiliary and cardiac systems, salivary glands, and thyroid. ^{99m}Tc-tetrofosmin is eliminated through the biliary system into the intestines, and through the renal system. At 48 hours 40% of the injected activity is eliminated via the kidneys and 26% via the bowel.[36]

Adverse Effects

Adverse effects are rare. Angina, hypertension, and torsades de pointes have been reported but probably occurred because of underlying heart disease. Other adverse effects include flushing, dyspnea, headache, vomiting, abdominal discomfort, metallic taste, burning sensation in the mouth, unusual odor, and mild leukocytosis.[6]

Contraindications

The only contraindication to ^{99m}Tc-tetrofosmin injection is hypersensitivity to any agent in the kit.

MTM Concerns

The FDA pregnancy category is C. Technetium, as free pertechnetate, crosses the placenta and is distributed into breast milk.[33] Based on ^{99m}Tc-sestamibi studies, breast-feeding should be interrupted for 4 hours.[11] Beta-blocking and calcium-channel-blocking medications often prevent the patient from achieving the desired heart rate and may reduce the sensitivity of the test. Depending on the clinical necessity or the clinical question, these agents may need to be discontinued by the patient's physician prior to examination for a time sufficient to obviate their pharmacologic effect. Patients should fast for at least 4 hours prior to exercise or pharmacologic stress.[30] Prolonged proton pump inhibitor therapy, but not H_2-receptor antagonist therapy, may contribute to stomach wall activity, affecting the diagnostic accuracy of the study.[37]

Carbon C 14 Urea

Carbon C 14 urea (^{14}C-urea) is used for in vitro testing to detect gastric urease indicating the presence of *Helicobacter pylori* (*H. pylori*) in the human stomach.[38] The test is not used often but has been recommended for documenting the eradication of *H. pylori* after treatment.

Dosage and Administration

The adult dosage of ^{14}C-urea in capsule form for oral administration is 1 mg urea labeled with 1 µCi of ^{14}C.[38]

The patient takes the capsule with 20 mL of warm water followed by an additional 20 mL of warm water. A sample of the patient's breath is then collected at 10 minutes.[38]

After ingestion of the capsule by a patient infected with *H. pylori*, ^{14}C excretion in the breath peaks between 10 and 15 minutes and declines thereafter with a biologic half-life of about 15 minutes. The ^{14}C-urea that comes into contact with *H. pylori* in the stomach is hydrolyzed into ^{14}C-carbon dioxide and ammonia. The carbon dioxide enters the bloodstream and is exhaled by the patient. ^{14}C-urea that is not hydrolyzed by *H. pylori* is excreted in the urine with a half-life of approximately 12 hours. About 10% of the ^{14}C remains in the body at 72 hours and is gradually excreted with a biologic half-life of 40 days.[38]

Adverse Effects

There are no known adverse effects with the use of ^{14}C-urea.

Contraindications

There are no known contraindications to the use of ^{14}C-urea.

MTM Concerns

Antibiotics, proton pump inhibitors, sucralfate, and bismuth preparations are known to suppress *H. pylori* and severely decrease the sensitivity of the test. Patients should not have had antibiotics or bismuth for 4 weeks. Patients should not have had proton pump inhibitors or sucralfate in the previous 2 weeks. Antacids and H_2-blockers do not affect the sensitivity of the test. If used to determine eradication, the test should be performed no sooner than 1 month after completion of therapy.[39] The medical use of ^{14}C-urea does not require a radioactive materials license.[40]

Gallium Citrate Ga 67

Gallium citrate Ga 67 (^{67}Ga-gallium citrate or ^{67}Ga-citrate) has been used in the past in a variety of tumor and inflammatory studies. It is indicated for the diagnostic imaging of Hodgkin's disease, lymphomas, bronchogenic carcinoma, and chronic inflammatory abscesses. ^{67}Ga-citrate is used most frequently for suspected recurrence of lymphoma and for monitoring the effects of therapeutic regimens.[1]

Dosage and Administration

The adult dosage of ^{67}Ga is 6–12 mCi administered intravenously. The pediatric dosage should be a fraction of the adult dosage based on the child's body size or weight.[41]

The gallium scan requires no preparation of the patient or the radiopharmaceutical. Imaging does not begin until approximately 24 hours after injection, to permit normal excretion of the radiopharmaceutical and clearance from the soft tissue. Because of its long half-life, imaging with gallium can continue up to 76 hours after initial injection if needed.[8] Imaging up to 96 hours has been performed to distinguish tumor from normal bowel accumulation that will clear over time.[1]

After intravenous injection, the citrate complex dissociates in the blood and ^{67}Ga becomes bound to plasma transferrin. Eighty-five percent of the ^{67}Ga activity has a biologic half-life of 25 days. Elimination from the body is slow, with 25% of the injected dose excreted by the kidneys in the first 24 hours and 35% by the kidneys and bowel at 7 days.[1] Normal localization is in the liver, spleen, GI tract, kidneys (renal cortex), skeleton, and bone marrow. Localization in these organs is nonspecific, and the exact mechanism of ^{67}Ga citrate localization in infection and tumors is not clear. The theory is that ^{67}Ga bound to transferrin passes into the leukocyte or tumor, where it binds to lactoferrin.

Adverse Effects

Adverse effects are rare, but occurrences of hypersensitivity reactions or allergic reactions, skin rash, and nausea have been reported in association with ^{67}Ga-citrate use.[42]

Contraindications

^{67}Ga-citrate has no known contraindications, but because of its benzyl alcohol content it should be administered with caution to newborns, particularly infants born prematurely, and individuals with impaired liver function. ^{67}Ga-citrate contains 9 mg/mL or 0.9% benzyl alcohol as a preservative.[42] Gasping syndrome was shown to significantly decrease when benzyl alcohol use was discontinued in very low birth weight (less than 1 kg) newborns (less than 1 month old) and those less than 27 weeks' gestational age.[43] A dose of 0.5 mCi 14 days after ^{67}Ga-citrate calibration would contain approximately 44 mg of benzyl alcohol. It would be prudent to avoid use in this patient group, but the decision should be made case-by-case after consideration of the risks and benefits.

MTM Concerns

Daily laxatives or enemas are recommended during the first week after injection until the final images are obtained, in order to cleanse the bowel of radioactive material and minimize the possibility of false-positive studies.[42] ^{67}Ga-citrate is excreted in breast milk. It has been recommended that nursing be stopped until the infant's ingested effective dose equivalent is below 100 mrem, which would be approximately 3 weeks after administration of ^{67}Ga-citrate. Because of the difficulty of maintaining the maternal milk supply for such an extended period of time, complete cessation of nursing is usually recommended.[9] Many drugs and conditions alter the distribution of ^{67}Ga-citrate; this should be considered in interpreting study results. The drugs include antineoplastics, iron, intravenous calcium gluconate, corticosteroids, glucocorticoids, doxorubicin, phenytoin, antibiotics, and amiodarone. Altered biodistribution can occur secondary to drug-induced nephritis caused by drugs such as allopurinol or nonsteroidal anti-inflammatory drugs and after radiation therapy.[9] Patients should not have contrast (x-ray, CT, or gadolinium) during the time period needed for the ^{67}Ga-citrate scan.[44]

Indium In 111 Pentetate

Indium In 111 pentetate (^{111}In-pentetate, ^{111}In-diethylenetriaminepentaacetic acid, or ^{111}In-DTPA [GE Healthcare]) is used in radionuclide cisternography to study the flow of cerebrospinal fluid (CSF) in the brain, especially to diagnose normal-pressure hydrocephalus. It is also used to localize CSF leaks, test the patency of CSF shunts, and detect and quantify CSF rhinorrhea. In infants, ^{111}In-DTPA has been used to evaluate CSF dynamics and patency of the cerebral ventricular system.[9] ^{111}In-DTPA has also been used for liquid gastric emptying studies when a dual-isotope study is preferred.

Dosage and Administration

The adult dosage for CSF evaluation is 500 µCi slowly administered intrathecally into the subarachnoid space of the lumbar spine, usually administered by an interventional radiologist. In dual-isotope liquid gastric emptying studies, 100 µCi is administered orally with 4 ounces of water.

After intrathecal injection, the radiopharmaceutical is diluted in the patient's CSF and travels with the CSF around the spinal cord and to the brain, where it is absorbed into the bloodstream and then excreted from the body. This process occurs slowly, and imaging occurs at least 4 hours and possibly not until 24 hours after injection of the radiopharmaceutical. Imaging may occur over 2 or 3 days to ensure adequate documentation of the physiologic transit of the CSF.[8]

After intrathecal administration, ^{111}In-DTPA diffuses to the basal cisterns within 2 to 4 hours and subsequently appears in the sylvian and cerebral cisterns.[9] In normal individuals, the radiopharmaceutical will ascend to the parasagittal region within 24 hours, with simultaneous partial or complete clearance of activity from the basal cisterns and sylvian regions. The radiopharmaceutical does not normally enter the cerebral ventricles. Approximately 65% of the administered dose is excreted by the kidneys within 24 hours, and this increases to 85% by 72 hours. Images are obtained 4 and 24 hours after administration. Imaging for CSF leaks may take place at 1–2 hours, and nasal packs (pledgets) are usually used to confirm the presence of CSF rhinorrhea.[45]

Adverse Effects

Adverse effects have been seen in less than 0.4% of patients and include aseptic meningitis and pyrogenic reactions.[9] Other reported adverse effects are nausea, vomiting, erythema, flushing, pruritus, hives/urticaria, cardiac arrest, hypertension, headache, and one death 20 minutes postinjection.[6]

Contraindications

There are no known contraindications to the use of ^{111}In-DTPA.

MTM Concerns

Extreme care must be exercised to ensure aseptic conditions for intrathecal injections.[45] The FDA pregnancy category is C. ^{111}In crosses the placenta and is slightly distributed into breast milk. Breast-feeding should be interrupted for 24 hours.[9] Renal impairment will increase the radiation dose to the patient. Acetazolamide may affect study results.[9]

Indium In 111 Oxyquinoline

Indium In 111 oxyquinoline (^{111}In-oxine [GE Healthcare]) is indicated for labeling of leukocytes for infection imaging.

Dosage and Administration

The adult dosage of ^{111}In-oxine-labeled leukocytes is 500 µCi. ^{111}In-oxine should be used in pediatric patients only after considering the use of technetium-labeled leukocytes. The pediatric dosage is based on a fraction of the adult activity, using BSA or weight or the formula 0.0075–0.015 mCi/kg with a minimum activity of 0.05 mCi.[14]

For infection imaging, approximately 60 mL of blood must be withdrawn from the patient for radiolabeling. Isolation of the WBCs, labeling time, and transportation to a nuclear pharmacy, if used, result in a 2–3 hour delay before the labeled radiopharmaceutical is ready for injection into the patient. Imaging with ^{111}In-labeled leukocytes does not begin until approximately 24 hours after injection.[8]

When incubated with leukocytes in vitro (free of plasma containing transferrin), the lipophilic ^{111}In-oxine passively diffuses into the leukocyte cell membrane. Intracellularly, the ^{111}In binds to cytoplasmic proteins, becoming trapped inside the cell, and the oxyquinoline diffuses back out of the cell. The labeled leukocytes are then reinjected to permit the imaging of inflammatory sites through the normal physiologic properties of leukocytes.[9] After intravenous administration of the labeled leukocytes, about 60% of the activity will distribute equally to the spleen and liver, with some activity in the bone marrow. Part of normal biodistribution is lung accumulation immediately after injection, with a biologic half-life of 15 minutes and almost no activity left in the lungs at 4 hours. The renal and bowel elimination of ^{111}In-oxine-labeled leukocytes is 1% of the injected dose in the first 24 hours.[46]

Adverse Effects

Reported adverse effects include fever, diffuse rash, pruritus, and hives/urticaria.[6]

Contraindications

There are no known contraindications to the use of ^{111}In-oxine.

MTM Concerns

The FDA pregnancy category is C. ^{111}In crosses the placenta and is slightly distributed into breast milk. Breast-feeding should be interrupted for 24 hours.[9] For imaging in pediatric patients, technetium-labeled leukocytes should be considered before ^{111}In-oxine-labeled leukocytes. Altered biodistribution of ^{111}In-oxine-labeled leukocytes can occur when the patient has had long-term antibiotic or corticosteroid treatment or is currently receiving total parenteral nutrition.[9]

Indium In 111 Capromab Pendetide

Indium In 111 capromab pendetide (^{111}In-capromab pendetide; ProstaScint [EUSA Pharma]) is indicated for use in patients with biopsy-proven and clinically localized prostate cancer who are at high risk for metastasis. It is also indicated for use in postprostatectomy patients with a high clinical suspicion of occult recurrent or residual prostate cancer.[47]

Dosage and Administration

The dosage is 0.5 mg of capromab pendetide labeled with 5–6 mCi of ^{111}In and administered intravenously over 5–20 minutes with vital signs monitored.

The dose is injected into the patient slowly over 5 minutes to reduce the probability of an adverse reaction. An initial set of single-photon emission computed tomography (SPECT) and planar images is acquired at 30 minutes after injection. Delayed images to demonstrate radiopharmaceutical localization may be acquired at 48, 72, 96, and 120 hours after radiopharmaceutical injection.

Capromab is an intact IgG murine monoclonal antibody that reacts with prostate-specific antigen (PSA). PSA is a glycoprotein expressed by the prostate epithelium. Capromab is conjugated by the manufacturer to a bifunctional chelating compound, GYK-DTPA (capromab pendetide).[47] After intravenous administration ProstaScint has a very slow clearance from the vasculature and a very small volume of distribution. The biologic half-life is 67 ± 11 hours, and approximately 10% of the administered activity is excreted renally within 72 hours. Normal activity is seen in the liver, spleen, and bone marrow. Normal activity has also been seen in the bowel, blood pool, kidneys, bladder, and genitalia.[47]

Adverse Effects

Adverse effects include anaphylaxis, increased bilirubin levels, hypotension, hypertension, injection site reactions, elevated liver enzymes (possibly due to tumor), pruritus, fever, rash, headache, myalgia, asthenia, burning sensation in thigh, shortness of breath, alterations of taste, and production of human antimouse antibodies (HAMA) by the recipient.[6]

Contraindications

ProstaScint is contraindicated in patients who are hypersensitive to the product or any other murine product.

MTM Concerns

The patient must complete bowel cleansing preparation before the 3-day imaging procedure.[8] ProstaScint can be used only by physicians who have completed specific training by the manufacturer in image interpretation; the program is called Partners in Excellence. The administration of a murine antibody may induce HAMA.[47] HAMA formation may interfere with diagnostic tests that employ murine-based immunoassay techniques, such as tumor-marker PSA. HAMA formation also may alter the biodistribution of murine-based diagnostic imaging agents or therapeutic agents.

Indium In 111 Pentetreotide

Indium In 111 pentetreotide (^{111}In-pentetreotide; Octreoscan [Covidien]) is an agent for the scintigraphic localization of primary and metastatic neuroendocrine tumors bearing somatostatin receptors.[48]

Dosage and Administration

The adult dosage is 10 µg pentetreotide labeled with 6 mCi of ^{111}In and administered intravenously. The pediatric dosage is 10 µg pentetreotide labeled with 0.14 mCi/kg ^{111}In with a minimum activity of 1 mCi.[39]

Imaging using ^{111}In-pentetreotide typically occurs at 4 and 24 hours after radiopharmaceutical injection to permit adequate time for radiopharmaceutical accumulation in areas of abnormality.[8]

^{111}In-pentetreotide is a conjugate of the bifunctional chelate DTPA and octreotide, a long-acting analogue of the human hormone somatostatin. ^{111}In-pentetreotide binds to somatostatin receptors throughout the body.[48,49] After intravenous administration ^{111}In-pentetreotide is cleared rapidly from the blood, with 30% of the administered activity remaining in the blood pool at 10 minutes. Normal biodistribution occurs in the pituitary gland, thyroid gland, spleen, liver, and urinary bladder. Elimination is almost entirely via the kidneys, with 50% of the administered activity recovered in the urine by 6 hours and 85% within 24 hours. Bowel excretion is only about 2% of the administered dose. The biologic half-life of ^{111}In-pentetreotide is 6 hours.[48]

Adverse Effects

Adverse effects have been reported in less than 1% of patients and include dizziness, headache, hypotension, changes in liver enzymes, joint pain, and nausea.[48]

Contraindications

^{111}In-pentetreotide is contraindicated in patients who have a hypersensitivity to ^{111}In-pentetreotide or octreotide.

MTM Concerns

Patients may use a bowel prep prior to imaging to facilitate visualization of the abdominal area.[50] Many precautions should be taken in ^{111}In-pentetreotide administration. In patients suspected of having insulinoma, an intravenous infusion of glucose should be available because of the potential for inducing severe hypoglycemia. ^{111}In-pentetreotide should not be administered together with total parenteral nutrition solutions. Patients receiving octreotide therapy should suspend the medication 48 hours before administration of the radiopharmaceutical. For patients taking Sandostatin LAR (octreotide depot formulation), ^{111}In-pentetreotide should be administered 3.5 to 4 weeks after the last administration of Sandostatin LAR (about 3 days before the monthly injection).[39] Delayed imaging may be necessary for patients with decreased renal function.

Iodine I 123 Sodium Iodide

Iodine I 123 sodium iodide (^{123}I-sodium iodide) is indicated for diagnostic studies of the thyroid.

Dosage and Administration

The adult dosage for a diagnostic thyroid function test is 100–400 μCi administered orally. The lower end of the range (100 μCi) is recommended for uptake studies alone, and the higher end (400 μCi) for thyroid imaging.[51] Pediatric dosages should be a fraction of the adult activity based on BSA or weight. The pediatric minimum dosage is 10 μCi for uptake studies and 50 μCi for thyroid imaging.[9] Imaging begins approximately 24 hours after oral administration of radioiodine. The scan consists of a set of three images, each taken for 10 minutes.[8]

The action of radioiodide is based on the accumulation and retention of iodine as required for the synthesis of thyroid hormones. Radioiodide is also concentrated in functioning papillary/follicular thyroid cancer and metastases. Radioiodide is readily absorbed from the GI tract. Normal distribution is in the choroid plexus, gastric mucosa, salivary glands, nasal mucosa, and lactating breast tissue. In the thyroid, radioiodide is removed from the blood by thyroid epithelial cells via active transport. In the follicular colloid tissue, the iodide is oxidized to iodine and bound to tyrosyl residues of thyroglobulin. Thyroid uptake is usually increased in hyperthyroidism and in goiters with impaired hormone synthesis. Uptake is usually decreased in hypothyroidism. In the euthyroid patient, 5%–30% of the administered activity is concentrated in the thyroid gland at 24 hours and has an effective half-life of 8 hours. The biologic half-life in the thyroid compartment for euthyroid patients is 80 days; for hyperthyroid patients it is 5–40 days. The normal range of urinary excretion in 24 hours is reported to be 37%–75% of the administered dose, varying with thyroid and renal function. Less than 2% of the administered activity is excreted via the bowel and salivary glands at 48 hours.[9,51]

Contraindications

Patients with a hypersensitivity to ^{123}I should not receive the product.

MTM Concerns

Patient preparation for all thyroid procedures is critical. Medications given to patients with thyroid conditions, along with some vitamins, foods, and iodinated contrast media, may alter radiopharmaceutical uptake. If an oral radiopharmaceutical is to be administered, the patient should not consume food or drink for at least 2 hours before and after radiopharmaceutical administration to ensure that the radiopharmaceutical does not bind to food. Radioiodide uptake could be decreased by recent intake of stable iodine in any form or use of thyroid hormone, antithyroid drugs, or amiodarone. The patient should not have had a diagnostic study with radiographic contrast media within 4 weeks of radioiodide administration. Lithium increases radioiodide uptake.[9] Antithyroid medications such as methimazole and propylthiouracil should be discontinued before administration of the ^{123}I capsule because they will interfere with uptake of the radiopharmaceutical.[52]

Iobenguane I 123

Iobenguane I 123 (^{123}I-iobenguane, ^{123}I *meta*-iodobenzlyguanidine sulfate, ^{123}I-mIBG; AdreView [GE Healthcare]) is indicated for use in the detection of primary or metastatic pheochromocytoma or neuroblastoma as an adjunct to other diagnostic tests.[53]

Dosage and Administration

For adults and pediatric patients weighing over 70 kg the recommended dose is 10 mCi administered intravenously over 1–2 minutes. For pediatric patients the dosage is weight based and a chart is supplied in the manufacturer's product information. The typical pediatric dosage is 5 mCi with a minimum pediatric dosage of 1 mCi.[53] Imaging is performed 18–24 hours postadministration.

After intravenous administration ^{123}I-mIBG is rapidly cleared from the blood and accumulates mainly in the liver and to a lesser degree in the lungs, heart, spleen, and salivary glands. Most ^{123}I-mIBG activity is excreted unaltered by the kidneys via glomerular filtration. In patients with normal renal function, 40%–50% of the administered activity is eliminated within 24 hours,[9] and 70%–90% of the administered dose is recovered unaltered in urine within 4 days. Only a small amount (<1%) of the administered activity is eliminated via the bowel.[53]

Adverse Effects

Adverse effects have been mostly isolated occurrences; they include dizziness, rash, pruritus, flushing, and injection site hemorrhage.[53]

Contraindications

^{123}I-mIBG is contraindicated in patients with a known hypersensitivity to iobenguane or iobenguane sulfate.

MTM Concerns

Thyroid protection with 130 mg potassium iodide or potassium perchlorate should be administered orally at least 1 hour before ^{123}I-mIBG administration and should continue for 6 days after administration.[1,53] ^{123}I-mIBG is FDA pregnancy category C. ^{123}I is excreted into human breast milk. The AdreView product information suggests that nursing women consider interrupting nursing for 10 half-lives or 6 days. Drugs that block norepinephrine uptake or deplete norepinephrine stores may decrease ^{123}I-mIBG uptake in neuroendocrine tumors. When medically feasible, these drugs should be discontinued for at least 5 biologic half-lives before ^{123}I-mIBG administration; examples include antihypertensives that deplete norepinephrine stores or inhibit reuptake (e.g., discontinue reserpine and labetalol 72 hours before); antidepressants that inhibit norepinephrine transporter function (e.g., discontinue amitriptyline and derivatives, imipramine and derivatives, and selective serotonin reuptake inhibitors 48 hours before), and sympathomimetic amines (e.g., discontinue phenylephrine, phenylpropanolamine, pseudoephedrine, and ephedrine 24 hours before).[9,53] The package insert also states that "AdreView contains benzyl alcohol, which may cause serious reactions in premature or low birth-weight infants," and that "safety and effectiveness have not been established in pediatric patients <1 month of age." AdreView contains 10.3 mg/mL benzyl alcohol.[53] Gasping syndrome was shown to significantly decrease when benzyl alcohol use was discontinued in very low birth weight (less than 1 kg) newborns (less than 1 month old) and those less than 27 weeks' gestational age.[43] It would be prudent to avoid use in this patient group, but the decision should be made case-by-case after consideration of the risks and benefits.

Ioflupane I 123

Ioflupane I 123 (^{123}I-ioflupane; DaTscan [GE Healthcare]) is used as a diagnostic aid for Parkinson's disease. It is indicated as an adjunct to other diagnostic evaluations (symptoms or signs) suggestive of dopaminergic neurodegeneration.[54]

Dosage and Administration

The adult dosage for visualization of dopamine transporter distribution within the nigrostriatal neurons using SPECT is 3–5 mCi via slow intravenous injection over not less than 20 seconds. Imaging takes place 3–6 hours postinjection.[54]

^{123}I-ioflupane has rapid blood clearance, and at 5 minutes about 5% of the administered activity is present in circulation. Brain activity is about 7% of the injected activity at 10 minutes and 3% at 5 hours. The striatal activity is about 30% of the whole brain activity. ^{123}I-ioflupane is eliminated 60% through the kidneys and 14% via the bowel by 48 hours.[54]

Adverse Effects

No serious adverse events have been linked to the administration of ^{123}I-ioflupane. The frequency of reported adverse events (headache, nausea, vertigo, dry mouth, and injection site pain) is less than 1%.[54]

Contraindications

The only contraindication for ^{123}I-ioflupane is known hypersensitivity to the active substance or any of the components or iodine.

MTM Concerns

^{123}I-ioflupane is a Schedule II controlled substance, so Drug Enforcement Administration and state board of pharmacy laws regarding the ordering, handling, storage, and disposal of Schedule II medications must be followed. The thyroid should be protected by giving the patient the equivalent of 100 mg of iodide as either potassium iodide solution or Lugol's solution or 400 mg of potassium perchlorate to block the thyroid from taking up any free iodine 123; this should be administered at least 1 hour prior to ^{123}I-ioflupane injection.[54] The ioflupane in this radiopharmaceutical binds to the dopamine transporter, so drugs with high affinity for the dopamine transporter may interfere with the images obtained. Patients' medication lists should be screened for amoxapine, amphetamine, benztropine, bupropion, buspirone, cocaine, mazindol, methamphetamine, methylphenidate, norephedrine, phentermine, phenylpropanolamine, selegiline, and sertraline.[54] ^{123}I-ioflupane is pregnancy category C. A risk–benefit analysis should be done to determine whether the use of ^{123}I-ioflupane is necessary for the patient. It is not known whether ^{123}I-ioflupane is excreted in breast milk, but iodine 123 is excreted in breast milk. It is recommended that nursing patients discontinue breast-feeding and pump and discard the breast milk for 6 days after injection of ^{123}I-ioflupane.

Thallous Chloride Tl 201

Thallous chloride Tl 201 (^{201}Tl-chloride) is used most frequently in myocardial perfusion imaging to assess coronary artery disease. It is also used to assess myocardium survival or viability in stable patients after acute myocardial infarction for possible reperfusion procedures. ^{201}Tl-chloride is used infrequently in parathyroid disorders and tumor imaging.

Dosage and Administration

The adult dosage of ^{201}Tl-chloride is 2–4 mCi for myocardial perfusion imaging and 3–5 mCi for tumor imaging. The pediatric dosage for tumor imaging is 30 μCi/kg with a maximum activity of 3 mCi.[9]

Imaging should begin within 10 minutes of ^{201}Tl-chloride administration because thallium is not fixed in the myocardium but redistributes, and imaging should be completed by 30 minutes after administration.[1]

^{201}Tl accumulates in the cells of the myocardium and other tissues in a manner analogous to that of potassium. The initial biodistribution of ^{201}Tl is primarily related to regional blood flow. Ischemic myocytes take up less ^{201}Tl than nonischemic myocytes in proportion to the relative change in blood flow. When administered intravenously, ^{201}Tl rapidly clears from the blood with normal distribution in the heart, liver, and to a lesser extent the renal and testicular systems. At 10 minutes after administration, 4% of the administered activity is in the heart. Elimination is slow, with only 4%–8% of the administered activity eliminated in the urine within 24 hours.[9] The biologic half-life is approximately 10 days.[1]

Adverse Effects

Adverse effects are rare but include allergic reactions, blurred vision, hypotension, nausea, and sweating. The vial stopper can contain latex and may cause allergic reactions in providers or patients who are sensitive to latex.[55]

Contraindications

There are no known contraindications to the use of ^{201}Tl.

MTM Concerns

^{201}Tl is distributed into breast milk. Drug interactions that have been reported to decrease ^{201}Tl accumulation in the heart include interactions with digitalis glycosides and intravenous propranolol. Food increases ^{201}Tl distribution to the abdomen, including the stomach, liver, spleen, and intestines, which may interfere with cardiac imaging.[9,55]

Xenon Xe 133

Xenon Xe 133 gas (^{133}Xe) is used for the evaluation of pulmonary function and for imaging the lungs. It has been used in the past for assessment of cerebral blood flow.

Dosage and Administration

The adult dosage of ^{133}Xe is 10–20 mCi administered by inhalation from a closed respirator system or spirometer that traps the exhaled ^{133}Xe. The minimum pediatric dosage is 2 mCi.[9,56]

Patients should have a chest x-ray within 24 hours of the lung scan.[57] When administered by inhalation, ^{133}Xe gas is distributed in the lungs in a manner similar to that of air and represents the regions of the lung that are aerated. Ventilation imaging is performed as patients inhale the radioactive xenon. Successive images are obtained while patients hold their breath (15–35 second single-breath-hold image) and during phases of breathing (4–5 minutes rebreathing and washout from lungs).[9]

^{133}Xe passes through the airways into the alveoli. Xenon diffuses easily, passing through cell membranes and exchanging freely between blood and tissue. ^{133}Xe passes into the pulmonary venous circulation via capillaries. Most of the ^{133}Xe that passes through the peripheral circulation returns to the lungs and is exhaled.[56] Clearance from the lungs is rapid, and in normal patients lung outlines are not seen 3–5 minutes after initiation of the washout phase.[58] Because xenon is lipid soluble, appearance of radioactivity has been noted in the liver during the washout phase of a ventilation study, especially in patients with fatty liver infiltration.[9]

Adverse Effects and Contraindications

There are no known contraindications to or adverse effects of ^{133}Xe.[56] Patients receiving total parenteral nutrition therapy will have the appearance of radioactivity in the liver.[16]

Radiopharmaceuticals Used for Therapy

Sodium Iodide I 131

Sodium iodide I 131 (^{131}I-sodium iodide) is indicated for both diagnostic studies of the thyroid (in microcurie amounts) and therapeutic applications for thyroid disorders such as hyperthyroidism and thyroid cancer (in millicurie amounts).

Dosage and Administration

The adult dosage for a diagnostic thyroid function test is 10–30 µCi orally. The dosage of ^{131}I-sodium iodide depends on the thyroid disorder and can range from a whole-body scan with 2–5 mCi to the treatment of thyroid carcinoma, in which the dosage could be 200 mCi. The dosage is administered orally in capsule or liquid form. There is no sterile pyrogen-free form currently commercially available for intravenous administration.

Imaging is not typically performed for ^{131}I-sodium iodide treatment of hyperthyroid patients. Imaging can be performed on thyroid cancer patients 2–3 days after administration of ^{131}I-sodium iodide to determine the dose of ^{131}I for treating the patient and to assess for metastatic disease.

The action of radioiodide is based on the accumulation and retention of iodine as required for the synthesis of thyroid hormones. Thyroid retention of any radioactive iodide permits quantification of organ uptake and imaging of anatomic distribution in thyroid tissue. Radioiodide is also concentrated in functioning papillary/follicular thyroid cancer and metastases. Radioiodide is readily absorbed from the GI tract. Normal distribution is largely to the thyroid and kidneys and to a lesser extent the choroid plexus, gastric mucosa, salivary glands, nasal mucosa, and lactating breast tissue. In the thyroid, radioiodide is removed from the blood by thyroid epithelial cells via active transport. In the follicular colloid tissue, the iodide is oxidized to iodine and bound to tyrosyl residues of thyroglobulin. Thyroid uptake is usually increased in hyperthyroidism and in goiters with impaired hormone synthesis. Uptake is usually decreased in hypothyroidism. The biologic half-life in the thyroid gland for euthyroid patients is 80 days; for hyperthyroid patients it is 5–40 days. The normal range of urinary excretion in 24 hours is reported to be 37%–75% of the administered dose, varying with thyroid and renal function. Imaging with millicurie amounts of ^{131}I is usually performed 18–24 hours after administration.[9,59]

Adverse Effects

Adverse events associated with sodium iodide include hypersensitivity reactions, radiation toxicities, and metabolic events. Immediate adverse reactions typically are related to hypersensitivity (e.g., anaphylaxis, rash, hives, and bronchospasm). Radiation adverse events related to the dose include the following: bone marrow depression, leukopenia, thrombocytopenia, acute leukemia, anemia, blood dyscrasia, chromosomal abnormalities, radiation sickness, and death. Delayed radiation toxicity includes radiation thyroiditis, gastritis, and sialadenitis. Metabolic adverse events include hypothyroidism and exaggerated hyperthyroidism due to radiation thyroiditis. Tenderness and swelling of the neck, pain on swallowing, sore throat, and cough may occur about the third day after treatment.

Contraindications

Radioiodide is contraindicated in pregnant women. Radioiodide crosses the placenta and may cause severe and irreversible hypothyroidism in the neonate. The fetal thyroid begins to concentrate iodine during the 12th week of gestation. Since the dosage is administered orally, patients with vomiting and diarrhea should not receive radioiodide.

MTM Concerns

The patient must have a negative pregnancy test and discontinue breast-feeding. The patient must be on a low-iodine diet for 10–14 days prior to ^{131}I-sodium iodide administration. Dietary sources of iodine include but are not limited to iodized salt, milk/dairy products, eggs, seaweed and kelp products, commercial bread with iodine conditioners, chocolate, iodine-containing vitamins, and red dye #3.[60] Patients must discontinue the use of all thyroid hormones unless recombinant human thyroid-stimulating hormone (rhTSH) is used.[60] Radioiodide uptake could be decreased by recent intake of stable iodine in any form or use of thyroid or antithyroid drugs or amiodarone. Lithium increases radioiodide uptake.[59] The patient should not have had a diagnostic study with radiographic contrast media within 4 weeks of radioiodide administration. No iodinated contrast media should be given to the patient within 3 months of ^{131}I therapy for cancer. Patients need to closely follow radiation safety precautions to avoid exposing family members and the public to radioactive iodine, for example, avoiding public transportation, sleeping in their own bed, using their own bathroom, minimizing time spent in close proximity to children and pregnant women, and using utensils that can be washed since throwing items contaminated with radioactive iodine in the trash may lead to alarm activation at landfills.

^{131}I-Tositumomab

^{131}I-tositumomab (Bexxar [Corixa and GlaxoSmithKline]) is indicated as a single-course treatment in patients with relapsed non-Hodgkin's lymphoma refractory to rituximab. This regimen should not be used as initial therapy.[61]

Dosage and Administration

Treatment with ^{131}I-tositumomab ("Bexxar therapeutic regimen") is a two-step regimen consisting of an initial "dosimetric" step to determine the patient dosage and, 7–14 days later, the "therapeutic" step. Both steps require a 450-mg predose of tositumomab in 50 mL of normal saline (0.9% sodium chloride) administered intravenously over 1 hour. In the dosimetric step, 5 mCi of ^{131}I-tositumomab in 30 mL of normal saline is administered intravenously over 20 minutes. The patient's therapeutic dosage is then based on the patient's elimination rate in the dosimetric step. If it is fast, then the therapeutic dosage of ^{131}I-tositumomab will be high. If the patient's elimination is slow, then the dosage of ^{131}I-tositumomab will be decreased. The treatment goal is to expose the lymphoma to 75 cGy of radiation (65 cGy if platelet count is below 150,000 cells/mm^3). The patient's dosage in the therapeutic step will depend on the information obtained from the dosimetric step.[61]

During administration, the same 0.22-μm in-line filter must be used for both the predose of tositumomab and the ^{131}I-tositumomab dosage.[61] Vials of ^{131}I-tositumomab may contain free iodine in the head space after thawing. A charcoal venting system is recommended to avoid airborne ^{131}I.

For the dosimetric portion of the treatment, the patient is imaged after urination on 3 different days to determine the elimination rate of ^{131}I-tositumomab.

Tositumomab is a murine monoclonal antibody directed against the CD20 antigen, which is found in high density on normal mature B lymphocytes and on greater than 90% of B-cell non-Hodgkin's lymphomas (NHLs). Tositumomab possesses all the cytotoxic properties of antibodies for cell death, namely, induction of apoptosis, complement-dependent cytotoxicity, and antibody-dependent cellular cytotoxicity. ^{131}I-tositumomab is a radioiodinated derivative of tositumomab that has been covalently linked to iodine 131. ^{131}I has beta-particle decay properties that result in localized therapeutic radiation and destruction of cells. The beta-particle effective path length in tissue is about 1 mm and can have cytotoxic effects on cells not reached by the antibody. This effect is called "crossfire."[1,61] The tositumomab administered as a predose before each step is given to decrease the spleen uptake and increase the terminal half-life of ^{131}I-tositumomab, thereby increasing the percentage available for NHL uptake. The median total-body effective half-life of ^{131}I-tositumomab, as measured by total-body gamma camera counts, in 980 patients with NHL was 67 hours (range, 28–115 hours).[61]

Adverse Effects and Contraindications

The Bexxar therapeutic regimen is contraindicated in patients with known hypersensitivity to murine proteins or any other component of the Bexxar regimen. Serious hypersensitivity reactions, including some with fatal outcome, have been reported during and after administration of the Bexxar therapeutic regimen. The regimen is contraindicated in patients with >25% lymphoma marrow involvement, platelet count <100,000 cells/mm^3, or neutrophil count <1,500 cells/mm^3. The most common adverse reactions associated with the regimen have been severe or life-threatening cytopenias. The time to nadir was 4–7 weeks and the duration of cytopenias was approximately 30 days. Because of the variable onset of cytopenias, complete blood counts should be obtained weekly for 10–12 weeks. Patients who have received murine proteins should be screened for HAMA. No formal drug interaction studies have been performed. Because of the frequent occurrence of severe and prolonged thrombocytopenia, the potential benefits of medications that interfere with platelet function or anticoagulation should be weighed against the potential increased risk of bleeding and hemorrhage. ^{131}I-tositumomab is pregnancy category X because iodine 131 may cause harm to the thyroid gland of the fetus.

MTM Concerns

Because of the risk of hypothyroidism, the patient must receive a thyroid-protecting agent such as saturated solution of potassium iodide (SSKI) before and after the ^{131}I-tositumomab infusion. The recommended dosing regimen is 4 drops of SSKI three times a day at least 24 hours prior to the infusion and continuing for 14 days posttreatment.[61] Also, before beginning the infusion of the nonradioactive tositumomab, 650 mg of acetaminophen and 50 mg of diphenhydramine are given to the patient orally. Patients should be counseled to use effective contraceptive methods throughout the treatment and for 12 months thereafter because of the potentially toxic effects on the male and female gonads.[61]

Samarium Sm 153 Lexidronam

Samarium Sm 153 lexidronam (^{153}Sm-lexidronam, ^{153}Sm-ethylenediaminetetramethylenephosphonic acid, or ^{153}Sm-EDTMP; Quadramet [EUSA Pharma]) is used for palliative treatment of bone pain from skeletal metastases. It is indicated for relief of pain in patients with confirmed osteoblastic metastatic bone lesions that enhance on radionuclide bone scan.[62]

Dosage and Administration

The adult dosage is 1 mCi/kg administered intravenously over 1 minute.[62]

Imaging is not typically performed, but if desired it can be done about 3 hours after injection of ^{153}Sm.

^{153}Sm decays by beta and gamma emission. The beta emissions of ^{153}Sm result in localized therapeutic radiation and destruction of cells. The exact mechanism of bone pain palliation is not known. ^{153}Sm-EDTMP has an affinity for bone and concentrates in bone metastases in a similar manner as the ^{99m}Tc-diphosphonate bone imaging agents and their association with hydroxyapatite cells.[1] ^{153}Sm-EDTMP clears rapidly from the blood, with 15% of the administered activity remaining at 30 minutes and 1% remaining at 5 hours after administration. Distribution is primarily to the sites of bone metastatic lesions and is about 65% of the administered activity. Elimination is renal, with approximately 35% of the administered activity excreted in the urine in 6 hours.

Adverse Effects and Contraindications

^{153}Sm-EDTMP is contraindicated in patients who have known hypersensitivity to EDTMP or similar phosphonate compounds. Because of the potential for bone marrow suppression, beginning 2 weeks after ^{153}Sm-EDTMP administration blood counts should be monitored weekly for at least 8 weeks or until recovery of adequate bone marrow function. Some patients have reported a transient increase in bone pain shortly after injection (flare reaction). This is usually mild and self-limiting and occurs within 72 hours of ^{153}Sm-EDTMP administration.[62]

MTM Concerns

The patient must have a complete blood count within 7 days of ^{153}Sm treatment to determine that the WBC and platelet counts are adequate to withstand treatment, since ^{153}Sm may lead to bone marrow suppression. Osteoblastic disease will need to be confirmed by a radionuclide bone scan within 3 months of the ^{153}Sm treatment. The patient should be well hydrated and should be encouraged to urinate frequently for the first 24 hours postadministration to reduce the radiation dose to the bladder.

Strontium Chloride Sr 89

Strontium chloride Sr 89 (^{89}Sr-chloride; Metastron [GE Healthcare]) is used for the palliative treatment of bone pain from skeletal metastases.

Dosage and Administration

The adult dosage of ^{89}Sr-chloride is 40–60 µCi/kg, with a maximum of 4 mCi administered intravenously over 1 to 2 minutes.[63]

Imaging is not performed.

^{89}Sr is a pure beta emitter. The beta emissions of ^{89}Sr result in localized therapeutic radiation and destruction of cells. The exact mechanism of bone pain palliation is not known. After intravenous administration, ^{89}Sr-chloride distributes similarly to calcium, clearing rapidly from the blood and selectively localizing in bone mineral. Uptake of strontium by bone occurs preferentially in sites of active osteogenesis in hydroxyapatite cells, not in bone marrow cells. The retained ^{89}Sr delivers a radiation dose sufficiently large to produce a palliative effect. Depending on the extent of disease, 12%–90% of the administered activity is distributed to metastatic bone lesions.[9] Elimination of the remaining activity is 66% renal and 33% via the bowel. Urinary excretion is highest in the first 48 hours after administration.[63]

Adverse Effects and Contraindications

^{89}Sr-chloride should not be used in patients with platelet counts below 60,000 cells/µL and white cell counts below 2,400/µL. It is recommended that the patient's peripheral blood cell counts be monitored at least once every other week for 3 to 4 months after ^{89}Sr administration. The nadir of platelet depression in most patients occurs between 12 and 16 weeks after administration, with return to preadministration levels 6 months after treatment. Repeated administrations of ^{89}Sr-chloride should be based on an individual patient's response to therapy, current symptoms, and hematologic status and are generally not recommended at intervals of less than 90 days.[63] A calcium-like flushing sensation has been observed in patients after rapid (less than 30-second) injection. A small number of patients have reported a transient increase in bone pain at 36–72 hours after injection. Saturation of bone binding sites by calcium medications may cause decreased uptake of ^{89}Sr-chloride. Calcium-containing products should be discontinued 2 weeks before and 2 weeks after administration of ^{89}Sr-chloride.[9]

MTM Concerns

The patient must have a complete blood count within 7 days of ^{89}Sr treatment to determine that the WBC and platelet counts are adequate to withstand treatment, since ^{89}Sr may lead to bone marrow suppression. Osteoblastic disease will need to be confirmed by performing a radionuclide bone scan within 3 months before the ^{89}Sr treatment. The patient should be well hydrated and should be encouraged to urinate frequently for the first 24 hours postadministration to reduce the radiation dose to the bladder.

Yttrium Y 90 and Indium In 111 Ibritumomab Tiuxetan

Yttrium Y 90 ibritumomab tiuxetan (^{90}Y-ibritumomab; "Zevalin therapeutic regimen" [Spectrum Pharmaceuticals]) is indicated as a single-course treatment in patients with relapsed non-Hodgkin's lymphoma refractory to rituximab.

Dosage and Administration

Treatment with ^{90}Y-ibritumomab is a two-step regimen consisting of an initial imaging step to determine the patient's localization of ibritumomab and, 7–9 days later, the treatment step. Both steps require a 250 mg/m^2 predose of rituximab administered intravenously at a rate of 50 mg/hr within 4 hours of the radiolabeled ibritumomab. In the imaging step, 5 mCi of ^{111}In-ibritumomab is administered intravenously over 20 minutes. In the treatment step, 0.4 mCi/kg of ^{90}Y-ibritumomab for patients with platelet counts exceeding 150,000/µL (0.3 mg/kg for platelet counts between 100,000 and 149,000/µL) up to a maximum dosage of 32 mCi is administered intravenously over 10 minutes.[64]

Imaging is performed 48–72 hours after ^{111}In-ibritumomab administration to assess for abnormal biodistribution of the radiopharmaceutical, which would cause the ^{90}Y-ibritumomab to be unsafe for the patient.

Ibritumomab is a murine monoclonal antibody directed against the CD20 antigen, which is found in high density on normal mature B lymphocytes and on greater than 90% of B-cell NHLs. Ibritumomab possesses all the cytotoxic properties of antibodies for cell death, namely, induction of apoptosis, complement-dependent cytotoxicity, and antibody-dependent cellular cytotoxicity. ^{90}Y-ibritumomab tiuxetan is a radiolabeled derivative of ibritumomab that has been covalently linked to yttrium 90. ^{90}Y is a pure beta emitter that results in localized therapeutic radiation and destruction of cells. The beta-particle effective path length in tissue is about 5 mm and can have cytotoxic effects on cells not reached by the antibody. This effect is called "crossfire."[1,64] ^{111}In-ibritumomab permits gamma camera imaging, performed at 24 and 48 hours, to confirm normal biodistribution of the antibody prior to treatment with ^{90}Y-ibritumomab. Abnormal distribution to the lung and kidney excludes treatment with ^{90}Y-ibritumomab. The mean effective half-life for ^{90}Y-ibritumomab activity in blood is 30 hours. Over 7 days, a median of 7.2% of the injected activity is excreted in urine.[64]

Adverse Effects and Contraindications

The Zevalin therapeutic regimen is contraindicated in patients with known type I hypersensitivity or anaphylactic reactions to murine proteins or to any component of this product, including rituximab, yttrium chloride, and indium chloride. The Zevalin therapeutic regimen should not be administered to patients with more than 25% lymphoma marrow involvement, a platelet count less than 100,000/µL, or a neutrophil count less than 1,500/µL or to patients with a history of failed stem cell collection. Severe cutaneous and mucocutaneous reactions have occurred with onset of 3 days to 4 months, including erythrema multiforme and Stevens-Johnson syndrome. ^{90}Y-ibritumomab should not be administered to patients with altered biodistribution of ^{111}In-ibritumomab. The Zevalin therapeutic regimen may cause severe, potentially fatal infusion reactions. These severe reactions typically occur during the first rituximab infusion, with time to onset of 30–120 minutes. Because the Zevalin therapeutic regimen includes the use of rituximab, the prescribing information contained in the package insert for that product should be followed except for dose. The most common severe adverse events reported with the Zevalin therapeutic regimen have been thrombocytopenia (61% of patients with platelet counts <50,000/µL) and neutropenia. For all patients, the median time to nadir was 7–9 weeks and the median duration of cytopenias was 22–35 days. Weekly monitoring for cytopenias and their complications (e.g., fever, neutropenia, hemorrhage) is necessary for up to 3 months after administration. Caution should be exercised in treating patients with drugs that interfere with platelet function or coagulation following the Zevalin therapeutic regimen. Patients who have received murine proteins should be screened for HAMA, which may alter ibritumomab biodistribution. The most common toxicities reported have been neutropenia, thrombocytopenia, anemia, GI symptoms (nausea, vomiting, abdominal pain, and diarrhea), increased cough, dyspnea, dizziness, arthralgia, anorexia, anxiety, and ecchymosis. The dosage of ^{90}Y-ibritumomab must not exceed 32 mCi regardless of the patient's weight. A 0.22-µm low-protein-binding filter should be in line between the syringe and the infusion port prior to injection of ^{111}In-ibritumomab and ^{90}Y-ibritumomab.[64]

MTM Concerns

The patient's platelet count must be determined on day 1 of the procedure to calculate the dose of ^{90}Y-ibritumomab. The patient is treated with diphenhydramine and acetaminophen prior to the rituximab infusion.

Conclusion

A radiopharmaceutical is used in every procedure performed in the nuclear medicine department. Radiopharmaceuticals are drugs that are subject to the same medication management standards as therapeutic medications. The goal of managing radiopharmaceuticals is to identify, resolve, and prevent any drug-related problem during the nuclear medicine procedure. Although the potential for an adverse reaction or a significant drug interaction exists with a nuclear medicine procedure, these events are not frequent. The overall prevalence of adverse reactions to radiopharmaceuticals has been documented at 2.3 per 100,000 administrations.[65] Of greater concern with radiopharmaceuticals is the possibility of a therapeutic drug or some other agent producing an unexpected alteration in the radiopharmaceutical's biodistribution, which may negatively affect the quality of the nuclear medicine study.[66]

References

1. Kowalsky RJ, Falen SW, eds. *Radiopharmaceuticals in Nuclear Pharmacy and Nuclear Medicine.* 2nd ed. Washington, DC: American Pharmacists Association; 2004
2. Neurolite [package insert]. Billerica, MA: Bristol-Myers Squibb Medical Imaging; 2003.

3. American College of Radiology. ACR practice guideline for the performance of single photon emission CT (SPECT) brain perfusion and brain death studies. 2007 (Resolution 21). www.acr.org/SecondaryMainMenuCategories/quality_safety/guidelines/nuc_med/ct_spect_brain_perfusion.aspx. Accessed September 2011.
4. Holman BL, Hellman RS, Goldsmith SJ, et al. Biodistribution, dosimetry, and clinical evaluation of technetium-99m ethyl cysteinate dimer in normal subjects and in patients with chronic infarction. *J Nucl Med.* 1989;30:1018–24.
5. Ziessman HA, O'Malley JP, Thrall JH. *Nuclear Medicine: The Requisites in Radiology.* Philadelphia: Elsevier Mosby; 2006.
6. Sampson CB. Adverse reactions and drug interactions with radiopharmaceuticals. *Drug Saf.* 1993;8:280–94.
7. American College of Radiology–Society for Pediatric Radiology. ACR-SPR practice guideline for the performance of adult and pediatric hepatobiliary scintigraphy. 2008 (Resolution 11). www.acr.org/SecondaryMainMenuCategories/quality_safety/guidelines/nuc_med/hepatobiliary_scintigraphy.aspx. Accessed September 2011.
8. Grantham V, Winn JM. Clinical applications of radiopharmaceuticals in the nuclear medicine department. In: Smith BT, ed. *Nuclear Pharmacy Concepts and Applications.* Gurnee, IL: Pharmaceutical Press; 2010.
9. *USP DI Volume I Drug Information for the Health Care Professional.* 19th ed. Englewood, CO: Micromedex; 1999.
10. Hepatolite [package insert]. Bedford, MA: Pharmalucence; 2008.
11. Harding LK, Bossuyt A, Pellet S, et al. Recommendations for nuclear medicine physicians regarding breastfeeding mothers. *Eur J Nucl Med.* 1995;22:BP17.
12. Society of Nuclear Medicine. Guideline for hepatobiliary scintigraphy. 2010. http://interactive.snm.org/docs/Hepatobiliary_Scintigraphy_V4.0b.pdf. Accessed September 2011.
13. Ceretec [package insert]. Arlington Heights, IL: GE Healthcare; 2006.
14. American College of Radiology–Society of Nuclear Medicine–Society for Pediatric Radiology. ACR-SNM-SPR practice guideline for the performance of scintigraphy for inflammation and infection. 2009 (Resolution 15). www.acr.org/SecondaryMainMenuCategories/quality_safety/guidelines/nuc_med/infections_inflammation.aspx. Accessed September 2011.
15. Laven DL, Clanton JA, Hladik WB III, et al. 2000. *Pharmacologic Alterations in the Biorouting/Performance of Radiopharmaceuticals Used in Nuclear Medicine.* Vol 1-4. Lenexa, KS: Gammascan Consultants; 2000.
16. Hladik WB III, Ponto JA, Lentle BC, et al. Iatrogenic alterations in the biodistribution of radiotracers as a result of drug therapy: reported instances. In: Hladik WB III, Saha GB, Study KT, eds. *Essentials of Nuclear Medicine Science.* Baltimore: Williams & Wilkins, 1987.
17. Pulmolite [package insert]. Bedford, MA: Pharmalucence; 2008.
18. American College of Radiology–Society of Nuclear Medicine–Society for Pediatric Radiology. ACR-SNM-SPR practice guideline for the performance of pulmonary scintigraphy in adults and children. 2009 (Resolution 13). www.acr.org/SecondaryMainMenuCategories/quality_safety/guidelines/nuc_med/pulmonary_scintigraphy.aspx. Accessed September 2011.
19. Choletec [package insert]. Princeton, NJ: Bracco; 2007.
20. American College of Radiology. ACR practice guideline for the performance of adult and pediatric skeletal scintigraphy (bone scan). 2007 (Resolution 20). www.

acr.org/SecondaryMainMenuCategories/quality_safety/guidelines/nuc_med/skeletal_scintigraphy.aspx. Accessed September 2011.
21. MDP-Bracco [package insert]. Princeton, NJ: Bracco Diagnostics; 2006.
22. Hesslewood S, Leung E. Drug interactions with radiopharmaceuticals. *Eur J Nucl Med.* 1995;21:348–56.
23. Patrick GM, Poznak CV, Modi S, et al. Intravenous bisphosphonate therapy does not acutely alter nuclear bone scan results. *Clin Breast Cancer.* 2010 (Feb):33–9.
24. MAG-3 [package insert]. St Louis: Mallinckrodt; 2005.
25. Society of Nuclear Medicine. SNM procedure guideline for diagnosis of renovascular hypertension. 2003. http://interactive.snm.org/docs/pg_ch16_0403.pdf. Accessed September 2011.
26. American College of Radiology–Society for Pediatric Radiology. ACR–SPR practice guideline for the performance of adult and pediatric renal scintigraphy. 2008 (Resolution12). www.acr.org/SecondaryMainMenuCategories/quality_safety/guidelines/nuc_med/renal_scintigraphy.aspx. Accessed September 2011.
27. HDP [package insert]. St Louis: Mallinckrodt; 2005.
28. DTPA Pharmalucence [package insert]. Bedford, MA: Pharmalucence; 2008.
29. Technelite [package insert]. Billerica, MA: Lantheus Medical Imaging; 2008.
30. American College of Radiology–Society of Nuclear Medicine–Society for Pediatric Radiology. ACR–SNM–SPR practice guideline for the performance of cardiac scintigraphy. 2009 (Resolution 14). www.acr.org/SecondaryMainMenuCategories/quality_safety/guidelines/nuc_med/cardiac_scintigraphy.aspx. Accessed September 2011.
31. PYP [package insert]. Bedford, MA: Pharmalucence; 2008.
32. Ultratag [package insert]. St Louis: Mallinckrodt; 2005.
33. Cardiolite [package insert]. Billerica, MA: Bristol-Myers Squibb Medical Imaging; 2003.
34. DMSA [package insert]. Arlington Heights, IL: GE Healthcare; 2004.
35. Sulfur colloid [package insert]. Bedford, MA: Pharmalucence; 2008.
36. Myoview [package insert]. Arlington Heights, IL: GE Healthcare; 2006.
37. Goel S, Bommireddipalli S, DePuey EG. Effect of proton pump inhibitors and H2 antagonists on the stomach wall in 99mTc-sestamibi cardiac imaging. *J Nucl Med.* 2009;37:240–3.
38. PYtest [package insert]. Draper, UT: Ballard Medical Products; 1997.
39. Balon HR, Roff E, Freitas JE, et al. SNM procedure guideline for C-14 urea breath test. Reston, VA: Society of Nuclear Medicine; 2002.
40. Exempt distribution of a radioactive drug containing one microcurie of carbon-14 urea. *Federal Register.* 1997;62(231):63634–40.
41. American College of Radiology–Society for Pediatric Radiology. ACR–SPR practice guideline for the performance of tumor scintigraphy (with gamma cameras). 2010 (Resolution 28). www.acr.org/SecondaryMainMenuCategories/quality_safety/guidelines/nuc_med/tumor_scintigraphy.aspx. Accessed September 2011.
42. Gallium 67-BMS [package insert]. Billerica, MA: Bristol-Myers Squibb Medical Imaging; 2005.
43. Hiller JL, Benda GI, Rahatzad M, et al. Benzyl alcohol toxicity: impact on mortality and intraventricular hemorrhage among very low birth weight infants. *Pediatrics.* 1986;77:500–6.
44. Shackett P. *Nuclear Medicine Technology: Procedures and Quick Reference.* 2nd ed. Philadelphia: Lippincott Williams & Wilkins; 2000.

45. Indium DTPA [package insert]. Arlington Heights, IL: GE Healthcare; 2006.
46. Indium oxine [package insert]. Arlington Heights, IL: GE Healthcare; 2006.
47. Prostascint [package insert]. Princeton, NJ: Cytogen; 1997.
48. Octreoscan [package insert]. St Louis: Mallinckrodt; 2006.
49. Intenzo CM, Fabbour S, Lin HC, et al. Scintigraphic imaging of body neuroendocrine tumors. *Radiographics.* 2007;27:1355–69.
50. Society of Nuclear Medicine. SNM practice guideline for somatostatin receptor scintigraphy V2.0. 2011. http://interactive.snm.org/docs/SRS_Final_V2_0.pdf. Accessed September 2011.
51. Sodium iodide I-123 capsules [package insert]. Arlington Heights, IL: GE Healthcare; 2005.
52. Society of Nuclear Medicine. SNM procedure guideline thyroid scintigraphy. 1999. http://interactive.snm.org/docs/pg_ch05_0403.pdf. Accessed September 2011.
53. Adreview [package insert]. 2008. Arlington Heights, IL: GE Healthcare; 2008.
54. DaTscan [package insert]. Arlington Heights, IL: GE Healthcare; 2011.
55. Thallium Lantheus [package insert]. Billerica, MA: Lantheus Medical Imaging; 2011.
56. Xenon 133 [package insert]. St Louis: Mallinckrodt; 2006.
57. Society for Nuclear Medicine. SNM practice guideline for lung scintigraphy V4.0. 2011. http://interactive.snm.org/docs/Lung_Scintigraphy_V4_Final.pdf. Accessed September 2011.
58. Saha GB, Swanson DP, Hladik WB III. Interventional studies in nuclear medicine. In: Hladik III WB, Saha GB, Study KT, eds. *Essentials of Nuclear Medicine Science.* Baltimore: Williams & Wilkins; 1987.
59. Sodium iodide 131 [package insert]. Kirkland, Quebec, Canada: Draximage; 2005.
60. Society of Nuclear Medicine. SNM procedure guideline for therapy of thyroid disease with iodine-131 (sodium iodide). http://interactive.snm.org/docs/Therapy%20of%20Thyroid%20Disease%20with%20Iodine-131%20v2.0.pdf. Accessed September 2011.
61. Bexxar [package insert]. Research Triangle Park, NC: GlaxoSmithKline; 2005.
62. Quadramet [package insert]. Princeton, NJ: Cytogen; 2003.
63. Metastron [package insert]. Arlington Heights, IL: GE Healthcare; 2006.
64. Zevalin [package insert]. Weston, MA: Biogen Idec; 2005.
65. Silberstein EB, Ryan J. Prevalence of adverse reactions in nuclear medicine. *J Nucl Med.* 1996;37:185–92.
66. Shaw SM. Diagnostic imaging and pharmaceutical care. *Am J Pharm Educ.* 1994; 58:190–3.

CHAPTER 7

Radiopharmaceuticals Used in Positron Emission Tomography Imaging

Kara D. Weatherman

Positron emission tomography (PET) imaging uses fairly short-lived, positron-emitting isotopes to produce three-dimensional images of functional processes that occur in the body. PET combines molecular biology and in vivo imaging, enabling cellular functions and metabolic processes within a living organism to be visualized without being significantly changed. An important advantage of PET imaging is that many of the isotopes that emit positrons are isotopes of common organic molecules such as carbon, nitrogen, oxygen, and fluorine. Thus, positron emitters can be incorporated into many different organic molecules with relative ease, which greatly enhances the clinical utility of this imaging modality.

Positron emission is a form of radioactive decay that occurs when the nucleus of an atom is proton rich. Within the nucleus, a proton is converted to a neutron, giving off a positron and a neutrino. A positron is a positively charged electron, carrying a positive 1 (1+) charge. The positron is released from the nucleus of the atom, but it is unable to exist for extended periods because it quickly collides with a negatively charged electron in the environment. The resulting annihilation reaction eliminates the positively and negatively charged particles, replacing them with two gamma photons. For this process to occur, a number of laws of conservation must be maintained. First, there must be conservation of electric charge. The net charge before the reaction (one positive, one negative) is zero. After the annihilation reaction, two uncharged gamma photons are created, resulting in a net charge of zero. Linear momentum and total energy must also be conserved. When the positron and electron annihilate, they produce two gamma photons, each with 511 keV of energy. When the collision occurs, the positron and electron have no net linear momentum, so the resulting photons are emitted in opposite directions (180°). The total energy of the system is equal to the rest energy of the electron and the positron (511 keV each). Positron emission can occur only if there is more than 1.022 MeV of excess energy in the system. If the energy difference is less than 1.022 MeV, the atom is unable to undergo positron decay, and decay will occur by electron capture.

In clinical use, the emission of the two 511-keV gamma photons allows PET imaging to take place. A PET camera consists of a ring of detectors that surround the patient. When a positron–electron annihilation occurs, the two 511-keV gamma photons travel in opposite directions and strike two detectors in the detector ring. The detectors are linked in circuit and, if both interactions occur within a short time window, the interactions are considered coincident. Interactions that do not "match" by falling within the requisite time are not recorded as true events. Coincidence detection enables a significant gain in sensitivity, allowing greater resolution and permitting smaller objects in the imaging field to be visualized.

Development of PET Imaging Agents

PET as an imaging modality can be traced back to experiments by scientists at the University of Pennsylvania, the Washington University School of Medicine, and Massachusetts General Hospital in the late 1950s.[1,2] At that time, the primary cyclotron-produced isotope in use was ^{15}O, which could be incorporated into $^{15}O_2$ gas, ^{15}O-CO_2, and ^{15}O-water. The availability of cyclotrons at the time was limited to government laboratories. However, by the mid-1970s biomedical facilities and universities began to have access to cyclotrons, and this led to greater availability of positron-emitting isotopes for clinical research. The development of ^{18}F-labeled 2-fluorodeoxy-D-glucose (^{18}F-FDG)[3] in the 1970s was the catalyst for the widespread expansion of PET as an imaging modality that has occurred since that time.

Table 7-1. Positron-Emitting Radioisotopes

Isotope	Half-life	Production
^{15}O (oxygen)	2 minutes	Cyclotron
^{13}N (nitrogen)	10 minutes	Cyclotron
^{11}C (carbon)	20 minutes	Cyclotron
^{18}F (fluorine)	110 minutes	Cyclotron
^{82}Rb (rubidium)	75 seconds	Generator
^{62}Cu (copper)	9.7 minutes	Generator
^{68}Ga (gallium)	68 minutes	Generator

Several positron-emitting isotopes are used clinically in nuclear medicine today (Table 7-1). The production of PET isotopes usually requires a cyclotron, which limits the availability of these isotopes to a predefined geographic distance from the production facility. However, generator-produced positron emitters may prove to be useful in expanding the geographic distribution of certain clinically useful isotopes.

The fairly short half-life of most positron-emitting isotopes serves as both a benefit and a hindrance to imaging. Short half-life isotopes decay quickly, decreasing the time that the radioactive isotope is retained in the body and thus decreasing the patient's exposure to radiation. The short half-life also allows administration of a greater amount of material (a larger dose), which can result in a higher-quality image. However, the short half-life can limit the clinical utility of the isotope.

Positron-emitting isotopes can be chemically manipulated and incorporated into other molecules to allow a greater range of clinical applications. The radiolabeled molecule, termed a radiopharmaceutical, will behave in the same manner as it would have before labeling, since the radioactive isotope simply replaces a nonradioactive atom of the molecule. Now, the localization and biodistribution of the molecule can be assessed by following the movement and localization patterns of the radioactive tracer. However, this is possible only if the chemical reactions required for the isotope substitution can be carried out in a reasonable time frame to ensure that sufficient quantities of radioactive material are present for imaging. With some PET isotopes, such as ^{15}O, with a 2-minute half-life, it is almost impossible to perform any appreciable chemical manipulation. However, isotopes such as ^{18}F, with a 110-minute half-life, can easily be incorporated into new compounds.

A short half-life can limit the availability of the isotope. For example, although ^{15}O-water is an excellent blood flow tracer, the 2-minute half-life of ^{15}O requires that a patient receiving it by infusion be in extremely close proximity to the cyclotron that produces it. Thus, the clinical use of this tracer is limited to facilities that have a cyclotron on site. In contrast, isotopes like ^{18}F that have a longer half-life can be produced and transported to users within a reasonable geographic distance. The material can be delivered by ground or air transportation to hospitals several hours away from the production facility.

Generator production offers the potential for easier distribution of short-lived imaging isotopes. Generator production requires a parent isotope (usually with a longer half-life) that will decay to form a daughter isotope (in this case, a positron-emitting isotope). When the generator is "eluted," the daughter isotope is removed from the generator, leaving the remaining parent isotope on the generator for further daughter production. The only commercially available PET generator system with Food and Drug Administration (FDA) approval for use, the ^{82}Rb generator for cardiac imaging, has a parent isotope (^{82}Sr) with a half-life of 25 days and a daughter isotope (^{82}Rb) with a half-life of 75 seconds.

Although PET radiopharmaceuticals have been available for more than 40 years, the production issues that have limited their applicability have also contributed to challenges in proving their clinical utility. This in turn has resulted in significant challenges with reimbursement that have further limited the clinical use of these agents. Historically, PET imaging has been limited to research. Although the *United States Pharmacopoeia (USP)* includes drug monographs for several PET radiopharmaceuticals, most PET radiopharmaceuticals have not been fully vetted through the FDA drug approval process. The FDA Modernization Act of 1997 required that FDA establish good manufacturing practices for PET drugs, which would include a dedicated approval path and separate standards for PET drugs than are used for other manufactured drugs. The standards, set forth in 21 CFR Part 212,

Current Good Manufacturing Practice (CGMP) for Positron Emission Tomography (PET) Drugs, determined that production of PET isotopes and related radiopharmaceuticals fell under the definition of manufacturing.[4] This regulation created a significant amount of controversy in the PET community because of the requirement that production of these agents be approved as a manufacturing process, which meant that any facility manufacturing PET radiopharmaceuticals would have to submit a new drug application (NDA) or an abbreviated new drug application (ANDA). As of August 2011, only four PET radiopharmaceuticals had been officially recognized by FDA through the traditional drug approval process (^{18}F-FDG, ^{18}F-sodium fluoride, ^{13}N-ammonia, and the ^{82}Sr–^{82}Rb generator).[5] Several cyclotron facilities throughout the United States have been involved in the production of PET radiopharmaceuticals under the scope of pharmacy compounding, but with the production of these materials now considered manufacturing, each facility must submit either an NDA or an ANDA to continue producing PET radiopharmaceuticals. The FDA final rule, published in December 2009, required all facilities to become compliant within 2 years (by December 2011).[4] Although these regulations will ensure that PET radiopharmaceuticals are of the highest quality, the increased cost of production and the legal requirements for compliance have the potential to affect the availability and the cost of these agents in the future.

PET Radiopharmaceuticals in Use

Although only four radiopharmaceuticals have FDA approval as drug entities, many other agents are used clinically in research settings throughout the country, and several of them have *USP* monographs. The research compounds are too numerous to cover in this chapter, but the FDA-approved agents are discussed here in detail.

^{18}F-2-Fluorodeoxy-D-Glucose (^{18}F-FDG)[6]

Indications

^{18}F-FDG is prepared by replacing one of the hydroxyl molecules on glucose with the ^{18}F molecule. ^{18}F-FDG acts as a glucose analogue in the body and is taken up by cells that have high glucose utilization. When administered by intravenous injection, ^{18}F-FDG is taken up by an active transport process via glucose transporters in the cell membrane in a manner analogous to glucose. However, once in the cell, the ^{18}F-FDG molecule is phosphorylated, effectively trapping it in the cell. The missing hydroxyl group prevents ^{18}F-FDG from being further metabolized. This allows the ^{18}F-FDG molecule to act as a marker of glucose utilization in the body. ^{18}F-FDG is most commonly used for imaging in the areas of neurology, cardiology, and oncology.

In the brain, glucose is the primary energy source, providing approximately 95% of the adenosine triphosphate (ATP) necessary for brain function. Because glucose metabolism is intimately connected with neuronal activity under physiologic conditions, it is an excellent marker for mapping neuronal activity.[7] Clinically, ^{18}F-FDG imaging allows visualization of areas of neuronal metabolic overactivity and underactivity. Increased metabolic activity is seen in tumors and in seizure foci during a seizure, and decreased metabolic activity may be present in conditions such as Alzheimer's disease.

In cardiology, ^{18}F-FDG can be used along with a blood perfusion tracer to evaluate myocardial viability. Traditional nuclear medicine blood perfusion tracers show the distribution of blood to areas of the myocardium. Decreased tracer deposition indicates a lack of blood flow to the area, either transient (ischemia) or permanent (infarction). Unfortunately, these types of tracers do not show the true metabolic capacity of the cells. The addition of ^{18}F-FDG allows further evaluation of the areas where there is a lack of blood flow during the perfusion portion of the study. If the tissue is infarcted (no longer viable), it will not take up ^{18}F-FDG. The area of interest will show no tracer uptake in either study (perfusion or metabolism), strengthening the diagnosis of infarction. In ischemia, blood flow to the area will be compromised and tracer uptake will be decreased in the tissues supplied by the blocked blood vessel. However, from a metabolic standpoint, the tissue is still viable and will still show ^{18}F-FDG uptake. The disparity between the two studies is a strong indicator that the tissue is still viable and that the patient will benefit from revascularization procedures to restore myocardial blood flow.

As an oncology agent, ^{18}F-FDG is useful in identifying rapidly proliferating tumor cells. Most cancers show rapid growth and require significant increases in both blood flow and metabolic fuel. Since many tissues use glucose as this fuel, the use of radiolabeled ^{18}F-FDG allows identification of areas of rapidly proliferating cells.

Following intravenous injection of ^{18}F-FDG, whole-body imaging can be performed to evaluate the location and extent of disease. ^{18}F-FDG imaging is used to identify primary lesions, stage disease by evaluating metastatic spread, monitor response to drug treatment, and evaluate disease recurrence. Although not all tumors are ^{18}F-FDG avid, the use of ^{18}F-FDG in oncology is currently the most common clinical use of this agent.

Dosage and Administration

^{18}F-FDG is often dosed by patient weight, with a usual dose between 5 and 15 mCi. After administration, the tracer is allowed to localize for approximately 45 minutes before imaging is started.

Adverse Reactions

Since ^{18}F-FDG is an analogue of a naturally occurring substance, adverse reactions are rare. In 1998, Silberstein and the Pharmacopeia Committee of the Society of Nuclear Medicine published a retrospective review of adverse reactions following 33,925 doses of PET radiopharmaceuticals, including the agents ^{18}F-FDG, ^{11}C-carbon dioxide, ^{11}C-methionine, ^{13}N-ammonia, and ^{15}O-water.[8] No adverse reactions to any of the agents in this study were reported.

Contraindications

There are no known contraindications to ^{18}F-FDG administration. Because of radiation issues, ^{18}F-FDG is a pregnancy category C drug and should be used with caution in pregnant women. Its excretion in breast milk has not been determined. ^{18}F-FDG has been used with increasing frequency in pediatric patients, although it has not been evaluated in this population.

Medication Therapy Management (MTM) Concerns

In most cases, administration of ^{18}F-FDG is dictated by the patient's glucose status. Glucose in the blood will compete with the ^{18}F-FDG for uptake in the tissues, so uptake of the radioactive tracer can be decreased in patients with elevated blood glucose levels in both neurologic and oncologic imaging studies. Ideally, studies in patients with and without diabetes should begin when glucose levels are euglycemic in order to maximize the uptake of the radioactive tracer. The patient's blood glucose should be checked upon presentation to the imaging department. Insulin administration to control blood glucose levels during neurologic and oncologic imaging is generally not recommended because it increases the possibility that the ^{18}F-FDG will be driven into muscle tissue, further decreasing the amount of tracer available for uptake in the desired location.[7,9]

In ^{18}F-FDG use for cardiac imaging, an inherent difficulty exists since the myocardium preferentially uses fatty acids for its metabolic needs unless there is an excess of glucose present or the myocardium is stimulated in some manner to take up the radioactive glucose agent. In patients without diabetes, an oral (25–100 mg) or intravenous glucose load is administered to ensure that the fasting blood glucose is greater than 250 mg/dL. Patients with blood glucose >250 mg/dL do not need glucose loading. Insulin is given according to the blood glucose level approximately 45–90 minutes after the oral glucose load. After administration of the ^{18}F-FDG, supplemental insulin is given to promote maximum uptake of the tracer in the normal myocardium. In diabetic patients who are less responsive to insulin, glucose loading may not work as well, and higher doses of insulin may be needed to achieve acceptable uptake of tracer in the heart tissue.[9,10]

In ^{18}F-FDG use for oncology imaging, many patients undergo a dual PET/CT scan. This allows for correlation of the metabolic activity map generated by the PET imaging procedure with the anatomic data obtained from the CT scan. To maximize the information obtained by the CT scan, most patients receive either intravenous or oral contrast during the CT phase of the study. Chapter 4 provides further information on x-ray contrast media.

^{18}F-Sodium Fluoride[11]

Indication

^{18}F-sodium fluoride is indicated as a bone imaging agent to define areas of altered osteogenic activity. ^{18}F-sodium fluoride was first approved by FDA as a bone imaging agent in 1972, but it fell out of favor when the ^{99m}Tc-labeled bone imaging agents became available in the mid-1970s. ^{18}F-sodium fluoride has been listed by FDA as a discontinued drug since 1984. Fluoride ions accumulate in the skeleton in relation to blood flow to the bone and the bone's efficiency in extracting fluoride ions from the blood. ^{18}F-sodium fluoride has a faster blood clearance and twofold higher uptake in bone than the currently available ^{99m}Tc-MDP imaging agent.[11] Increased uptake of the ^{18}F-sodium fluoride tracer is seen in areas of arthritis, trauma, fracture, various diseases of the skeletal system, and primary and metastatic malignancy in the bone, as well as in rapidly growing epiphyses in children.

Dosage and Administration

In its original FDA approval, ^{18}F-sodium fluoride had a recommended dosing range of 0.5–2 mCi with a maximum dose of 4 mCi. However, current recommendations for dosing range from 5 mCi to 10 mCi. Obese patients may need a dose at the higher end of this range. Pediatric administration is based on weight (0.06 mCi/kg), with a minimum recommended activity of 0.5 mCi and a maximum activity of 5 mCi.[12] Compared with ^{99m}Tc agents, ^{18}F-sodium fluoride has a high bone-to-soft-tissue ratio, rapid localization in the skeleton, and rapid clearance from the blood circulation, so imaging can begin as soon as 30–45 minutes after injection and as soon as 90 minutes for whole-body or extremity imaging.[12] Because of tracer clearance by the renal system, imaging with the ^{99m}Tc agents requires a 2–3 hour delay between injection and imaging to improve the bone-to-soft tissue ratio.

Adverse Reactions

Since fluoride is a normal body constituent, few adverse effects would be expected after the administration of this agent. An FDA review in 2000 found no reports of adverse reactions to ^{18}F-sodium fluoride administration; this was based on reports of adverse reactions from the original NDA (0/400 patients) and review of the published literature.[13]

Contraindications

There are no known contraindications to the administration of ^{18}F-sodium fluoride. As with any radioactive imaging agent, use in pregnancy should be avoided unless the benefit to the mother exceeds the potential risk of radiation exposure of the fetus.

MTM Concerns

No patient preparation is required for an ^{18}F-sodium fluoride bone scan. Patients do not need to fast, nor do they need to discontinue current medications before the study. The effect of diphosphonate drug therapy on ^{18}F-sodium fluoride bone uptake has not been studied, but since these drugs have not been shown to affect studies with the traditional ^{99m}Tc bone imaging agents, it is likely that they also will not affect ^{18}F-sodium fluoride bone scans.[14,15] To minimize radiation dose to the bladder since the agent will be excreted renally, patients should be encouraged to drink two or more 8-ounce glasses of water 1 hour prior to injection and two or more after administration of the tracer.[11]

^{13}N-Ammonia

Indication

^{13}N-ammonia is a myocardial perfusion tracer that is rapidly cleared from the blood into the myocardial tissue in proportion to myocardial blood flow.[16] It is trapped in the myocardium because the radionuclide is incorporated into glutamine in the cells via glutamine synthetase.[17] In August 2007 FDA approved an NDA for this agent submitted by the Feinstein Institute for Medical Research in New York.[18] In myocardial perfusion imaging, both stress and rest studies can be performed to map perfusion patterns to determine ischemic or infarcted tissues.

Dosage and Administration

The normal dose of ^{13}N-ammonia for both rest and stress imaging is 10–20 mCi administered as an intravenous bolus. Imaging can be started 3 minutes after the injection since the biologic half-life is 2.84 minutes in the blood and less than 2 minutes in the myocardium.[19] A second study can be performed approximately 40 minutes after the first study is completed.

Adverse Reactions

No adverse reactions after ^{13}N-ammonia administration have been reported.[8]

Contraindications

There are no known contraindications to the administration of ^{13}N-ammonia.[19]

MTM Concerns

Like most radiopharmaceuticals, ^{13}N-ammonia carries a pregnancy category C designation. It is not known if ^{13}N-ammonia is excreted in breast milk, but it is recommended that after administration to breast-feeding women, alternative nutrition sources for the infant should be used for 2 hours, which is more than 10 half-lives of the drug. The safety of this agent in pediatric patients has not been established. Patients receiving this radiopharmaceutical, which is excreted renally, should be encouraged to drink plenty of fluids and void frequently to minimize radiation dose to the bladder.

^{82}Rb-Chloride

Indication

^{82}Rb-chloride is an injectable PET imaging agent used to evaluate regional myocardial perfusion during both rest and stress conditions in adults with suspected or existing coronary artery disease. ^{82}Rb-chloride is a potassium analogue and is extracted from the blood by the myocardium via the sodium–potassium ATPase ion pump present in the cell membrane. ^{82}Rb is taken up in viable myocardium; it is cleared rapidly from infarcted tissues. The presence of infarction or ischemia can be noted as early as 2 minutes after administration and is seen as photon-deficient cold areas in the myocardium.[20] ^{82}Rb-chloride is available as a generator system because of the short (75-second) half-life of the isotope. The generator system was first approved in 1989.[21]

Dosage and Administration

Since ^{82}Rb has such a short half-life, administration of the radiopharmaceutical requires a direct infusion of the tracer as the generator is being eluted. The normal adult dose is 40 mCi, with a range of 30–60 mCi, and should be infused at a rate of 50 mL/minute. Since the half-life is short, it is possible to perform both rest and stress studies in the same day. If a second study is ordered, the activity of the second dose would be the same as the first. The maximum total volume for all studies performed should not exceed 100 mL. For rest imaging, acquisition begins within 60 seconds of the infusion and lasts approximately 5 minutes. Stress images can be started within 10 minutes of the first imaging study.[21]

Adverse Reactions

No adverse reactions to the administration of ^{82}Rb-chloride have been reported in published literature or postmarketing experience reports.

Contraindications

There are no known contraindications to the administration of ^{82}Rb.

MTM Concerns

^{82}Rb-chloride is listed as a pregnancy category C drug, and its excretion in human milk is not known. With the short half-life of ^{82}Rb, it is unlikely that any drug would be excreted in human milk. To ensure that no radioactive material is present in the milk, breast-feeding should be withheld for 1 hour after the last infusion of the drug. The use of this agent in pediatric patients has not been studied. Since this agent is used in patients with cardiac issues and the radiopharmaceutical is administered in large volumes, transitory increases in volume load may be induced in patients with congestive heart failure; patients should be observed for several hours after administration to ensure that no hemodynamic alteration has occurred. This is especially important with elderly patients, and consideration should be given to increasing the time between rest and stress images to help reduce fluid load between studies.[21]

USP Monographs

USP drug product monographs provide information that is useful during product compounding and preparation, including standards for ensuring stability and purity of the final products. Over the years, *USP* has included monographs for several commonly used PET radiopharmaceuticals that have not been officially approved as drug products by FDA. If these drugs continue to be used, they will need to go through a formal NDA or ANDA process.[4] The PET imaging agents that have *USP* monographs are listed in Table 7-2.

Table 7-2. PET Drugs with *USP* Monographs

^{18}F-Fludeoxyglucose Injection
^{18}F-Fluorodopa Injection
^{18}F-Sodium Fluoride Injection
^{11}C-Carbon Monoxide
^{11}C-Flumazenil Injection
^{11}C-Mespiperone Injection
^{11}C-Methionine Injection
^{11}C-Raclopride Injection
^{11}C-Sodium acetate injection
^{13}N-Ammonia Injection
^{15}O-Water

Research

Research into the development of new PET tracers will continue to expand, given their ability to be incorporated into a variety of drug molecules and their advantages such as short radioactive half-life, use in real-time imaging of biodistribution, and acquisition of high-resolution images. Several promising radiopharmaceuticals are currently undergoing clinical investigation.

Conclusion

PET imaging is often considered the future of nuclear medicine. The ability to incorporate PET isotopes into a variety of compounds, the short half-life of the isotopes, and the wide range of applications will allow this imaging modality to maintain its important role in patient management. Furthermore, these imaging agents are extremely safe, and their administration will produce few if any problems.

References

1. Ter-Pogossian M, Phelps M, Hoffman E, et al. A positron emission transaxial tomography for nuclear imaging (PETT). *Radiology.* 1975;114:89–98.
2. Phelps M, Hoffman E, Mulani N, et al. Application of annihilation coincidence detection to transaxial reconstruction tomography. *J Nucl Med.* 1975;16:210–24.
3. Ido T, Wan C-N, Casella V, et al. Labeled 2-deoxy-D-glucose analogs—labeled 2-deoxy-2-fluoro-D-glucose, 2-deoxy-2-fluoro-D-mannose and C-14-2-deoxy-2-fluoro-D-glucose. *J Labelled Comp Radiopharm.* 1978;14:175–82.
4. US Food and Drug Administration. Current good manufacturing practice (CGMP) for positron emission tomography (PET) drugs. 21 CFR Part 212.
5. US Food and Drug Administration. FDA approved drug products. www.accessdata.fda.gov/scripts/cder/drugsatfda/index.cfm. Accessed September 2010.
6. Fludeoxyglucose F-18 Injection [package insert]. New York: Citigroup Biomedical imaging Center, Weill Medical College of Cornell University; 2004.
7. Society of Nuclear Medicine. Procedure guideline for FDG PET brain imaging. Version 1.0. 2009. http://interactive.snm.org/docs/Society%20of%20Nuclear%20Medicine%20Procedure%20Guideline%20for%20FDG%20PET%20Brain%20Imaging.pdf. Accessed September 2010.
8. Silberstein E. Prevalence of adverse reactions to positron emitting radiopharmaceuticals in nuclear medicine. *J Nucl Med.* 1998;39:2190–2.
9. Society of Nuclear Medicine. Procedure guideline for tumor imaging with ^{18}F-FDG PET/CT. Version 1.0. 2006. http://interactive.snm.org/docs/jnm30551_online.pdf. Accessed September 2010.
10. American Society of Nuclear Cardiology. Cardiac F-18 FDG PET practice points. www.asnc.org/imageuploads/PP-PETFDG081511.pdf. Accessed August 2011.
11. Cancer Imaging Program, Division of Cancer Treatment and Diagnosis. Sodium fluoride F 18 injection investigator's brochure. Bethesda, MD: National Institutes of Health; 2008. http://imaging.cancer.gov/images/documents/Generic-NaF_IB_Edition1_10-2009.pdf. Accessed August 2011.
12. Society of Nuclear Medicine. Procedure guideline for sodium ^{18}F-fluoride PET/CT bone scans. Version 1.0. Reston VA: Society of Nuclear Medicine; 2010. http://

interactive.snm.org/docs/Procedure_Outline_NaF_PETV1.0.pdf. Accessed September 2010.
13. Food and Drug Administration. Positron emission tomography drug products: safety and effectiveness of certain PET drugs for specific indications. *Federal Register.* 2000(Mar 10);65:12999–13009.
14. Percherstorfer M, Schillhing T, Jjanisch S, et al. Effect of clodronate treatment on bone scintigraphy in metastatic breast cancer. *J Nucl Med.* 1993;34:1039–44.
15. Carrasquillo J, Whatley M, Dyer V, et al. Alendronate does not interfere with 99mTc-methylene diphosphonate bone scanning. *J Nucl Med.* 2001;42:1359–63.
16. Shah A, Schelbert HR, Schwaiger M, et al. Measurement of regional myocardial blood flow with N-13 ammonia and positron emission tomography in intact dogs. *J Am Coll Cardiol.* 1985;5:92–100.
17. Moerlein SM. Radiopharmaceuticals for positron emission tomography. In: Kowalsky RJ, Falen SW, eds. *Radiopharmaceuticals in Nuclear Pharmacy and Nuclear Medicine.* Washington, DC: American Pharmacists Association; 2004:346.
18. Food and Drug Administration. Ammonia N-13 drug detail. www.accessdata.fda.gov/scripts/cder/drugsatfda/index.cfm?fuseaction=Search.DrugDetails. Accessed September 2010.
19. Ammonia N-13 injection prescribing information. Manhasset, NY: Feinstein Institute for Medical Research. January 2011. www.accessdata.fda.gov/drugsatfda_docs/label/2011/022119s001lbl.pdf. Accessed August 26, 2011.
20. CardioGen Rb-82 Injection [package insert]. South Plainfield, NJ: Bracco Diagnostics; 2010. www.accessdata.fda.gov/drugsatfda_docs/label/2010/019414s012lbl.pdf. Accessed September 2010.
21. Food and Drug Administration. Rubidium-82 drug detail. www.accessdata.fda.gov/scripts/cder/drugsatfda/index.cfm?fuseaction=Search.DrugDetails. Accessed September 2010.

CHAPTER 8

Adjunct Agents Used in Nuclear Medicine Imaging

Nonradioactive Pharmaceuticals

Vivian S. Loveless

Nuclear medicine imaging is noninvasive and provides valuable information on functional processes within the body. In order to enhance the information gleaned or shorten the time for imaging, interventional agents are frequently used as an adjunct in select studies. Unlike radiopharmaceuticals, these agents do possess pharmacologic activity, so they do present a greater risk for adverse events. Pharmaceutical care for a patient undergoing a nuclear medicine study that uses an interventional agent includes screening for potential drug interactions before the study and monitoring for adverse events during and after the procedure. If an adverse event occurs, it is critical to know the treatment. This chapter describes the use of interventional agents, categorized according to the type of imaging.

Brain Imaging

Acetazolamide

When patients have suffered transient ischemic attacks and the computed tomography (CT) scan is normal, single-photon emission computed tomography (SPECT) can be used to demonstrate an abnormality.

However, without pharmacologic intervention, most cerebral cortical perfusion defects are not demonstrated. When cerebrovascular disease, including carotid stenosis, results in reduced blood flow to the brain, autoregulatory compensatory vasodilation distal to the stenotic site maintains the oxygen supply. This is the mechanism for the cerebrovascular reserve. Acetazolamide provides a means of assessing the capacity of the cerebrovascular reserve.[1]

Mechanism of Action

Acetazolamide is a potent enzyme inhibitor acting particularly on carbonic anhydrase, which is an enzyme responsible for catalyzing the reversible reaction involving the dehydration of carbonic acid and hydration of carbon dioxide.[2] By increasing the level of CO_2, acetazolamide causes a vasodilatory response in normal cerebral blood vessels.[3]

Dosage and Administration

This radiopharmaceutical study is carried out in two stages: one with acetazolamide and one without (baseline). The order of the stages varies between institutions.[4,5] A sample protocol is for 1 gram of acetazolamide to be intravenously administered over 2 minutes, after which the patient is monitored for 25 minutes for adverse events, including blood pressure changes. Twenty minutes after administration of acetazolamide, the radiopharmaceutical is administered.[5]

Medication Therapy Management (MTM) Concerns

Some patients have experienced light-headedness, a short-acting diuretic effect, and paresthesias around the mouth and in the distal limbs.[6] It has also been noted that adverse reactions common to sulfonamide derivatives may arise.[7] Cross-reactivity between sulfonanamide-based drugs has remained controversial. Sulfonamides can be divided into three groups based on their chemical structure (sulfonylarylamines, nonsulfonylarylamines, and sulfonamide moiety not directly attached to a benzene ring). Acetazolamide falls into the nonsulfonylarylamine category. Johnson et al.[8] performed a comprehensive review of the literature regarding sulfonamide cross-reactivity; they concluded that the data do not support sulfonylarylamine cross-reactivity with nonsulfonylarylamines. Using a database in the United Kingdom, Strom et al.[9] conducted a retrospective cohort study regarding the safety of sulfonamide nonantibiotics in patients having had prior allergic reactions to sulfonamide antibiotics. Their results revealed an association between hypersensitivity after sulfonamide antibiotic administration and subsequent allergic reaction after receiving a sulfonamide nonantibiotic. However, they stated that the association seemed to be the result of a predisposition to allergic reactions rather than cross-reactivity between sulfonamide-based medications. The use of acetazolamide in patients with chronic, noncongestive angle-closure glaucoma and in those with hypersensitivity to acetazolamide is contraindicated.[7]

Cardiac Studies

Pharmacologic stress agents are used as an alternative to exercise stress in nuclear cardiology patients who are unable to exercise for medical reasons, such as those who have orthopedic impediments, elderly or deconditioned patients, and those with peripheral vascular disease and claudication. In addition, many patients are unmotivated and refuse to complete the test using exercise. Pharmacologic stress is used in patients receiving chronotropic agents (β-blockers or calcium-channel antagonists) because these medications may decrease the sensitivity of exercise-stress nuclear medicine scintigraphy.[10] Two types of pharmacologic stress agents are available for nuclear cardiology studies: vasodilators and inotropic/chronotropic agents.[11] The disparity in blood supply between ischemic and nonischemic vessels can be induced by pharmacologic stress agents.[12]

Adenosine

Mechanism of Action

Adenosine is a potent coronary vasodilator except in coronary vessels that are stenosed.[13] It has been postulated that adenosine produces its pharmacologic action through activation of cell surface receptors, specifically, the A_1 and A_2 adenosine receptors. The exact mechanism by which adenosine relaxes vascular smooth muscle is unknown. However, evidence exists supporting both activation of adenylate cyclase via smooth muscle cells' A_2 receptors and restraint of slow inward calcium current, resulting in decreased calcium uptake. Adenosine may also reduce vascular tone by adjusting sympathetic neurotransmission. A specific transmembrane nucleoside transport system mediates adenosine's intracellular uptake. After adenosine enters the cell, adenosine kinase quickly phosphorylates it to adenosine monophosphate, or adenosine deaminase deaminates it to inosine. Neither of these metabolites is vasoactive.[14] Even though adenosine's onset of action is much quicker than that of dipyridamole, the level of vasodilation is similar, leading to a 3-fold to 5-fold increase from baseline blood flow.[15]

Dosage and Administration

The recommended dosage regimen for adenosine is 0.140 mg/kg/min intravenously infused for 6 minutes, resulting in a total dosage of 0.84 mg/kg.[14] At 3 minutes (midpoint of infusion of adenosine), the myocardial perfusion radiopharmaceutical is intravenously administered.[15] It is necessary to monitor the patient's blood pressure, heart rate, and electrocardiogram (ECG).[10] Based on adenosine's kinetics, a 4-minute protocol with ^{201}Tl has been used in many institutions for more than 10 years. Reductions in time, cost, and side effects are all advantages of this protocol. The American Society of Nuclear Cardiology imaging guidelines have suggested that reasonable precedent has been set for this protocol.[16]

MTM Concerns

Adenosine administration is contraindicated in patients having unstable angina, critical aortic stenosis, hypertrophic obstructive cardiomyopathy, and recent onset of acute myocardial infarction (less than 24 hours).[17] Also, the use of adenosine is contraindicated in patients with second- or third-degree atrioventricular (AV) block (except in those with a functioning artificial pacemaker), those with a known or suspected bronchospastic or bronchoconstrictive lung disease, those with systolic blood pressure of less than 90 mm Hg (systemic hypotension), and those with a known adenosine hypersensitivity.[11,14]

Since dipyridamole potentiates adenosine's effects and side effects, dipyridamole should not be administered for 12–24 hours before the adenosine infusion.[15] Pharmaceuticals and foods containing methylxanthines (e.g., theophylline, caffeine) antagonize the effects of adenosine, so these must be withheld for 24 hours prior to the study.[13] Compared with dipyridamole, the first pharmacologic stress agent, adverse reactions to adenosine are more common, reportedly occurring in 75% of patients.[15] The three most common adverse reactions are flushing, chest discomfort, and dyspnea or urge to breathe deeply. These events normally require no treatment and are transient. A rare but more serious adverse event is AV block, usually occurring in the first few minutes of infusion; this effect is also transient.[15] About 6.3% of patients have been reported to experience AV block after adenosine injection, with first-degree and second-degree AV blocks more common than third-degree AV block.[14] To reverse the effects of adenosine, usually all that is necessary is terminating the infusion, since the serum half-life is less than 10 seconds.[13] Theophylline, in the form of aminophylline (50–125 mg by slow intravenous infusion) was required to abort side effects of adenosine in fewer than 2% of patients enrolled in controlled clinical trials in the United States.[14]

Dipyridamole

Mechanism of Action

Dipyridamole inhibits the reabsorption and metabolism of endogeneous adenosine. With a dipyridamole infusion, the biologic half-life of endogeneous adenosine is increased, resulting in tripling or quadrupling of the level of circulating natural adenosine. The elevated level of endogeneous adenosine causes the desired coronary hyperemia in normal vessels.[18] Upon administration of dipyridamole, stenosed vessels exhibit no further vasodilation, since they are at maximum dilation as a result of autoregulatory mechanisms activated by myocardial hypoperfusion. Thus, normal myocardial vessels exhibit proportionally elevated flow, whereas blood flow in the diseased vessels is not increased as much, depending on the level of stenosis.[15] Myocardial perfusion imaging in combination with dipyridamole can detect the disparity in regional blood flow between normal and abnormal coronary arteries.[18]

Dosage and Administration

The recommended dosage for dipyridamole as an adjunct to radionuclide myocardial perfusion imaging is 0.142 mg/kg/minute (total of 0.57 mg/kg) intravenously injected over 4 minutes. According to clinical experience, a dose greater than 60 mg is not necessary.[19] Monitoring of the blood pressure, ECG, and heart rate is necessary since these can be adversely affected by dipyridamole.[20] Three to four minutes after dipyridamole administration, the radiopharmaceutical is injected.[18]

MTM Concerns

Precautions must be considered in patients with unstable angina or recent myocardial infarction. Bronchospasm can be produced as a result of increased adenosine levels elicited by dipyridamole infusion.

Dipyridamole stress testing should not be performed in patients with systemic hypotension (systolic blood pressure <90 mm Hg), acute asthma, severe chronic obstructive pulmonary disease, or recent respiratory failure.[11,18] Since xanthine-containing pharmaceuticals (theophylline or aminophylline) can reverse dipyridamole's cardiovascular effects, Mettler and Guiberteau[15] recommend withholding these agents for 48 hours if patient toleration permits. However, Strauss et al.[11] advise against using vasodilator agents in any patients requiring methylxanthine pharmaceuticals to control their bronchospasm. Food containing a xanthine (e.g., caffeine) should be withheld for 24 hours prior to dipyridamole testing.[13]

In the event of severe bronchospasm or severe chest pain, aminophylline should be given by slow intravenous injection, using an initial dose of 50–100 mg over 30–60 seconds, with total doses ranging from 50 mg to 250 mg. Sublingual nitroglycerin can be given if aminophylline 250 mg does not relieve chest pain within a few minutes. The possibility of myocardial infarction should be taken into account if chest pain persists despite the administration of aminophylline and nitroglycerin. In a clinical study involving 3911 patients, the most frequently reported adverse events were chest pain/angina pectoris, ECG changes, headache, and dizziness.[19] Aminophylline is routinely administered in some clinics at the end of the dipyridamole stress study to prevent and alleviate common adverse effects of dipyridamole.[13]

Dobutamine

Mechanism of Action

Dobutamine is a synthetic catecholamine with β_1-agonist activity. It acts in a similar manner to exercise in that myocardial oxygen demand is increased via increases in both myocardial contractility and heart rate, and at higher doses there is an increase in systolic blood pressure that also increases the demand for oxygen.[15] Dobutamine at higher doses may also evoke heterogeneous myocardial blood flow distribution by increasing coronary blood flow in normal vessels by 1.5 to 2 times with less elevation in stenosed vessels. This difference can be demonstrated with myocardial perfusion imaging. Coronary blood flow increases less with dobutamine than with the vasodilators adenosine and dipyridamole. The increase in blood flow produced by dobutamine is similar in magnitude to that produced by exercise.[21]

Dosage and Administration

The dobutamine protocol varies between clinics. One protocol, for example, begins with intravenous administration of dobutamine at 5 µg/kg/min for 3 minutes, increasing to 10, 20, 30, and 40 µg/kg/min for each successive 3-minute period if tolerated by the patient.[13] The patient's ECG, heart rate, and blood pressure should be monitored throughout the infusion and should continue to be monitored after cessation of the infusion until symptoms subside and vital signs return to baseline.[12] After the maximum tolerated dose of dobutamine is achieved, the radiopharmaceutical is administered, with the dobutamine infusion continuing for at least 1 minute.[13]

MTM Concerns

Dobutamine is contraindicated in patients with acute myocardial infarction, uncontrolled hypertension, aortic stenosis, acute coronary syndromes, dissecting aneurysms, and any other conditions that could be worsened by the effects of this pharmaceutical.[22] Caution should be used in administering dobutamine to patients with atrial tachycardia.[15] Adverse effects have been reported in 75% or more of patients.[12] However, the most frequent adverse effects are transient; these include palpitations, chest pain, flushing, headache, and dyspnea.[15]

Dobutamine's biologic half-life is approximately 2 minutes, so a rapidly acting β-blocker is necessary in the event of a rare, persistent adverse event.[15] Esmolol, an intravenous β_1-blocker, can be used as an antidote, with a loading dose of 0.5 mg/kg/min for 1 minute, then 0.05 mg/kg/min for 4 minutes.[23] However, most drug-related adverse effects routinely resolve in 5–10 minutes after cessation of the infusion.[12]

With a dobutamine protocol, some patients may require atropine in order to increase the heart-rate response, even though this increase in heart rate does not produce the same augmentation in coronary blood flow as seen with a similar increase in heart rate evoked by exercise.[11] The intravenous dosage of atropine for this additional increase in heart rate is 0.5–1 mg.[24]

Regadenoson

Mechanism of Action

Coronary artery adenosine-mediated vasodilation entails activating the adenosine cyclase signaling pathway by way of the coronary endothelium's adenosine receptor.[22] Various subtypes of adenosine receptors have been discovered in different tissues. A_1 adenosine receptors are located in the AV node and are also responsible for renal vasoconstriction, whereas A_{2A} adenosine receptors are concentrated on the arterial vascular smooth muscle cells' surface. A_{2B} receptors play a role in peripheral vasodilation and bronchoconstriction, and the A_3 receptor is also involved in bronchoconstriction.[17] The hyperemic effects involved in coronary artery vasodilation are the result of activation of A_{2A} adenosine receptors.[22] Administration of regadenoson results in augmentation of blood flow in normal coronary arteries and little to no increase in stenotic coronary arteries.[25] Regadenoson is a selective A_{2A} adenosine-receptor agonist, so it offers a better side-effect profile than adenosine or dipyridamole, which both produce nonselective stimulation of all four subtypes of adenosine receptors.[17]

Adenosine and regadenoson have different pharmacodynamic profiles. With regadenoson, there is a 2-fold to 3-fold increase in myocardial blood flow, and this phase exhibits a half-life ranging from 2 to 4 minutes. The next phase has a half-life of 30 minutes on average, with a slow decrease in the pharmacodynamic effect. The last phase demonstrates a plasma half-life of about 2 hours.[17]

Dosage and Administration

Regadenoson's recommended dose is 0.4 mg given intravenously over approximately 10 seconds. Immediately after injection of regadenoson, a 5-mL saline flush should be injected. Ten to twenty seconds after the saline flush, the radiopharmaceutical is injected; the same catheter can be used for both injections.[25] For a minimum of 6 minutes after regadenoson injection, patients should be monitored.[17]

MTM Concerns

Since methylxanthines are nonspecific adenosine-receptor antagonists, there is potential for them to interfere with regadenoson's vasodilatory activity. Thus, it is recommended that for a minimum of 12 hours before regadenoson administration, patients refrain from consuming any products containing methylxanthines or taking any medications containing theophylline. Since dipyridamole may alter regadenoson's effects, it is advisable to withhold dipyridamole for a minimum of 2 days before the injection of regadenoson.[25]

Regadenoson is contraindicated in patients having second- or third-degree AV block or sinus node dysfunction unless a functioning artificial pacemaker is in place. Administration of this agent results in augmentation of blood flow in normal coronary arteries and little to no increase in stenotic coronary arteries.[25] Caution should be used in administering regadenoson to patients with chronic obstructive pulmonary disease or asthma. The most common adverse effects of regadenoson are dyspnea, headache, rhythm or conduction abnormalities, flushing, and angina or ST-segment depression.[17]

Regadenoson is comparable to adenosine for the identification of reversible myocardial perfusion defects, as was demonstrated in the Adenoscan Versus Regadenoson Comparative Evaluations for Myocardial Perfusion Imaging (ADVANCE-MPI). Regadenoson was better tolerated by patients in these trials. Even though the patients receiving regadenoson reported more headaches and gastrointestinal (GI) discomfort, they had a decreased rate of flushing and chest pain.[17] For the attenuation of persistent or severe adverse events, aminophylline may be administered.[25]

Endocrine Studies

Dexamethasone

When patients with hyperaldosteronism or hyperandrogenism are being evaluated with ^{131}I-6β-iodomethyl-19-norcholesterol (NP-59) scintigraphy, it is recommended that adrenocorticotrophic hormone (ACTH) secretion be suppressed in order to suppress NP-59 uptake at the site of cortisol production (zona fasciculata).[26] In the absence of suppression, interpretation of radiopharmaceutical uptake in the zona retucularis or zona glomerulosa would be quite complicated because of the normal high uptake in the zona fasciculata.[27]

Mechanism of Action

Dexamethasone suppresses the release of ACTH from the pituitary.[26]

Dosage and Administration

The dexamethasone suppression regimen consists of 4 mg of dexamethasone orally in divided doses beginning 7 days before the administration of NP-59 and continued until the end of the imaging sequence. Visualization of normal adrenal cortices is not expected for a minimum of 5 days after radiopharmaceutical administration.[26]

MTM Concerns

Patients who have a fungal infection or have ever had a hypersensitivity reaction to dexamethasone should not take dexamethasone. Also, patients receiving dexamethasone should avoid alcohol consumption and should take the medication with food in order to decrease stomach upset.[28] The literature should be consulted for a detailed list of drug interactions and other contraindications/precautions with this medication.

Potassium Iodide

Since the thyroid gland will take up radioactive iodide, potassium iodide is used as a radioprotective agent. Free radioiodide can be present when radiopharmaceuticals labeled with radioactive iodine are administered. This can be due to either in vivo degradation of radioiodinated radiopharmaceuticals or the presence of free radioiodide as a radiochemical impurity in the product itself.[26] Uptake of free radioiodide could cause unnecessary radiation exposure of the thyroid gland and potential misinterpretation of the images.

Mechanism of Action

When increased circulating stable (nonradioactive) iodides are present, they compete with the trapping and organification of radioiodine. Potassium iodide is administered to prevent uptake and organification of radioiodide, thus decreasing radiation dose to the thyroid gland.[26,29]

Dosage and Administration

For adrenocortical scintigraphy with NP-59, Thrall et al.[27] recommend that thyroid blocking begin at least 1 day before radiopharmaceutical administration and continue for 7 days, using the dosage regimen of 1 drop of saturated solution of potassium iodide (SSKI) (or its equivalent) given orally three times a day. The package insert for iobenguane I 123 (^{123}I-iobenguane) states that the radiation dose to the thyroid gland needs to be reduced by preventing uptake of free ^{123}I.[30] To block the thyroid gland in adults, it recommends administering 100 mg of

Table 8-1. Potassium Iodide Preparations[27,31]

Formulation	Potassium Iodide Content
Lugol's solution	130 mg/0.8 mL
SSKI[a]	38 mg/drop
Potassium iodide tablets	130 mg/tablet (equivalent to 100 mg iodine)
Potassium iodide tablets	65 mg/tablet (equivalent to 50 mg iodine)

[a]Saturated solution of potassium iodide.

iodide orally a minimum of 1 hour before radiopharmaceutical administration; the dosage for children should be adjusted according to body weight. Table 8-1 lists iodide preparations.

MTM Concerns

In patients with hypersensitivity to iodine, the use of potassium iodide is contraindicated.[32] When potassium iodide is given to a patient receiving other potassium-containing pharmaceuticals or potassium-sparing diuretics, a potential drug interaction exists. The result could be hyperkalemia and associated adverse events such as cardiac arrhythmias or cardiac arrest.[29]

Potassium Perchlorate

Swanson et al.[26] and the iobenguane I 123 package insert[30] recommend potassium perchlorate as an alternative to potassium iodide as a thyroid-blocking agent.

Mechanism of Action

Potassium perchlorate inhibits the selective thyroid uptake and concentration of iodide; this is thought to be a result of competitive inhibition of the thyroid's active transport system.[33]

Dosage and Administration

Potassium perchlorate is administered orally.[34] As an alternative to potassium iodide for blocking the thyroid, the package insert for iobenguane I 123 recommends an adult dosage of potassium perchlorate 400 mg administered at least 1 hour before radiopharmaceutical administration. For children, the dosage should be adjusted for body weight.[30]

MTM Concerns

When potassium perchlorate is administered, adequate amounts of water should be ingested to avoid gastric irritation.[34] Most adverse reactions to this agent are related to dose. In the past, potassium perchlorate was used as an antithyroid drug for hyperthyroidism at doses greater than 1000 mg daily, and the following adverse events were reported: gastric irritation, nausea, vomiting, pancytopenia, leukopenia, agranulocytosis, and fatal aplastic anemia.[33]

Recombinant Human Thyroid-Stimulating Hormone (rhTSH, Thyrotropin Alfa)

In contrast to normal thyroid tissue, thyroid cancer cells have a lower degree of radioiodine uptake.[31] It is desirable to have an elevated serum thyroid-stimulating hormone (TSH) level to maximize the sensitivity of detection of thyroid cancer with radioiodine imaging and to maximize the effectiveness of ^{131}I ablation of thyroid remnants in patients who have had total or near-total thyroidectomy. An elevated TSH level is also advantageous in palliative or curative radioiodine therapy of metastatic thyroid cancer. For many years, withdrawal of thyroid hormone was used to elevate endogenous TSH; this could require patients to be off their thyroid medication for up to 6 weeks. Patients would then frequently experience symptoms of hypothyroidism that would negatively affect their lives. The administration of rhTSH for the purpose of elevating TSH levels is an alternative to cessation of the exogenous thyroid hormone; the rhTSH method allows the patient to maintain adequate symptom control and bypass the symptoms of hypothyroidism. The use of rhTSH has been shown in several studies to be as efficacious as thyroid hormone withdrawal in the identification and ablation of a thyroid remnant.[35]

Mechanism of Action

When rhTSH is administered, it binds to TSH receptors located on normal thyroid epithelial cells or well-differentiated thyroid cancer cells, stimulating iodine uptake and organification along with synthesis and secretion of thyroglobulin (Tg), triiodothyronine (T3), and thyroxine (T4). This product has the same properties as endogenous thyrotropin and generates equivalent effects. Since the sialic acid content of rhTSH is higher than that of endogeneous pituitary TSH, there is lower in vitro bioactivity but greater in vivo potency associated with slower clearance.[36]

Dosage and Administration

The current recommendation is to intramuscularly administer 0.9 mg of rhTSH every 24 hours for 2 days,[36] with administration of the radioiodine 24 hours after the last injection of rhTSH.[35]

MTM Concerns

Some of the adverse events occurring after administration of thyrotropin alfa include atrial arrhythmias, hyperthyroidism, nausea, vomiting, hypersensitivity reactions, dizziness, headache, insomnia, paresthesia, and fatigue.[36] In clinical trials involving either single administration or repeated use of this agent, there were no reports of patients developing antibodies to thyrotropin alfa.[37]

Hepatobiliary Imaging

Sincalide (Cholecystokinin, CCK)

The secretion and release of endogeneous cholecystokinin from the duodenal mucosa is initiated upon the ingestion of a meal containing fat.[38,39] Cholecystokinin causes contraction of the gallbladder and relaxation of the sphincter of Oddi simultaneously. Also, there is an increase in intestinal motility along with inhibition of gastric emptying.[39] There are multiple clinical indications for CCK administration as an adjunct to hepatobiliary imaging or cholescintigraphy. When a patient has been fasting for more than 24 hours, the bile in the gallbladder becomes viscous and concentrated, preventing radiopharmaceutical entry. Administration of sincalide causes the gallbladder to contract and empty, which allows entry of the radiopharmaceutical.[38,40] Other clinical indications are the following: diagnosis of dysfunction of the sphincter of Oddi, differentiation between common-duct obstruction and functional causes, ruling out acute acalculous cholecystitis (if gallbladder fills), diagnosis of chronic acalculous cholecystitis, and diagnosis of chronic calculous cholecystitis.[38]

Mechanism of Action

Sincalide is the synthetic C-terminal octapeptide of cholecystokinin; it reproduces all the known biologic activities of endogeneous cholecystokinin.[39] Sincalide causes the gallbladder to contract, with evacuation of bile in a manner similar to that caused by endogeneous cholecystokinin. When sincalide is administered as a bolus dose, there is quick gallbladder contraction that becomes maximal in 5–15 minutes, in contrast to gallbladder contraction after a fatty meal, in which there is progressive contraction with maximal effects after about 45 minutes.[41]

Dosage and Administration

Protocols and dosages for the use of sincalide vary. One protocol calls for the administration of 0.02 μg/kg of body weight administered over 1–3 minutes by slow intravenous push.[38,42] Although 0.02 μg/kg is the dosage used most frequently, the administered dosage has ranged from 0.01 to 0.04 μg/kg among various clinics and institutions. In up to one-third of normal subjects, it has been demonstrated that the commonly used 0.01–0.02 μg/kg sincalide infusions given over 1–3 minutes produced unsuccessful gallbladder contractions. By using slower infusions (30–60 minutes) in these same subjects, effective contraction of the gallbladder was achieved.[38]

MTM Concerns

Adverse events of sincalide administration are usually transient and mild, with the most frequent being abdominal discomfort or pain and nausea. When this agent is administered very rapidly in a dose of 0.04 μg/kg, transient abdominal cramping is to be expected. These adverse reactions are commonly physiologic demonstrations of the drug's action, such as increased intestinal motility and delayed gastric emptying. These reactions can occur in normal patients as well as those with hepatobiliary disease. Other reported adverse events include dizziness, vomiting, flushing, rash, sweating, hypertension, hypotension, urge to defecate, shortness of breath, numbness, headache, diarrhea, and sneezing. These reactions can be diminished by using a lower infusion rate.[41]

Morphine

In a nuclear medicine hepatobiliary study, more time is needed to visualize a gallbladder in patients with increased intraluminal gallbladder pressure due to highly viscous stagnant bile. This time can be reduced with morphine-augmented cholescintigraphy, which provides as high a degree of accuracy as is obtained with conventional hepatobiliary imaging.[43] Morphine is used during a hepatobiliary scan when the gallbladder is not visualized by 60 minutes after radiopharmaceutical administration, to aid in the differentiation between acute and chronic cholecystitis.[38]

Mechanism of Action

Intravenous morphine increases the tone in the sphincter of Oddi and enhances intraluminal common bile duct pressure. The increased pressure within the common bile duct lumen is sufficient to overcome the increased bile flow resistance in a functionally obstructed, sludge-containing gallbladder and permit the radiopharmaceutical to enter the gallbladder if the cystic duct is not blocked.[43] If the gallbladder is visualized following morphine administration, this confirms that there is no blockage in the cystic duct and rules out acute cholecystitis. If the gallbladder fails to be visualized, the diagnosis of acute cholecystitis is confirmed.[44]

Dosage and Administration

The usual intravenous dose of morphine sulfate is 0.04 mg/kg of body weight diluted in 10 mL of 0.9% sodium chloride injection (normal saline), and administration is over 2–5 minutes.[44] In some departments, 2 mg is administered regardless of body weight.[42]

MTM Concerns

Patients usually tolerate this dosage well without major aggravation of symptoms.[44] If the effects of morphine need to be reversed, naloxone hydrochloride can be used. Morphine is contraindicated in patients with an allergy to morphine or with a history of pancreatitis.[42]

Phenobarbital

Hepatobiliary imaging has been used for many years to aid in the differentiation of biliary atresia from other causes of neonatal jaundice. Neonatal biliary atresia is characterized by the absence of intrahepatic and extraheptic bile ducts and inflammatory sclerosis.[38] The treatment for biliary atresia involves surgery, whereas neonatal hepatitis is self-limiting and is managed medically.[43]

Mechanism of Action

Phenobarbital activates liver excretory enzymes.[38] Its ability to stimulate bile production has been postulated to be a result of phenobarbital's action on the whole hepatic transport system for organic anions, independent of its effect on the hepatic enzymes.[45]

Dosage and Administration

The dosage that has achieved success is 5 mg/kg given orally in two divided doses for 5 days before administration of the radiopharmaceutical.[43]

MTM Concerns

To verify that a therapeutic level of phenobarbital has been achieved, it is recommended that the serum level be checked prior to the radiopharmaceutical study.[38]

Heterotopic Gastric Mucosa (Meckel's Diverticulum)

The most common and clinically significant type of heterotopic gastric mucosa is Meckel's diverticulum. In 10% to 30% of patients with Meckel's diverticulum, heterotopic gastric mucosa exists. Of these patients, about 60% are symptomatic, with 98% of this group experiencing bleeding.[46] Interventional agents are used to enhance the sensitivity of Meckel's diverticulum scintigraphy.[47]

Glucagon

Mechanism of Action

Glucagon's antiperistaltic effect is the result of relaxation of the smooth muscles in the GI tract.[47] The benefit of the antiperistaltic action is that it increases the persistence of radioactivity at the site of the diverticulum.[48]

Dosage and Administration

The glucagon dosage is 0.05 mg/kg administered intravenously 10 minutes after injection of ^{99m}Tc-pertechnetate.[47]

MTM Concerns

Few adverse effects have been seen with glucagon administration. Occasionally, nausea and vomiting may occur, as well as allergic reactions causing respiratory distress and hypotension. Symptomatic treatment is used for the adverse reactions.[49]

Histamine H_2 Antagonists

Mechanism of Action

Cimetidine and ranitidine are H_2-receptor antagonists that block secretion of ^{99m}Tc-pertechnetate from gastric mucosa cells into the gastric lumen.[46,47,49] The result is continued accumulation of the radiopharmaceutical within the gastric mucosa, with little movement into the intestinal tract. This effect greatly facilitates the visualization of the small area of Meckel's diverticulum.[49]

Dosage and Administration

Both of these agents are administered prior to ^{99m}Tc-pertechnetate administration. The adult oral dosage of cimetidine is 300 mg four times a day for 2 days, and the pediatric dosage is 20 mg/kg per day for 2 days (neonatal dosage 10–20 mg/kg per day). As an alternative to the oral route, cimetidine 300 mg in 100 mL of 5% dextrose injection can be given intravenously over 20 minutes. Imaging commences 1 hour later.[47]

The adult oral dosage of ranitidine is 150 mg, and the pediatric oral dosage is 2 mg/kg. The intravenous dosage of ranitidine is 1 mg/kg for infants, children, and adults, with a maximum dosage of 50 mg. Intravenous ranitidine is administered over 20 minutes, and imaging commences 1 hour later.[47]

MTM Concerns

A history of hypersensitivity reaction to cimetidine or any of its components is a contraindication to its use.[50] Relatively few adverse effects are associated with cimetidine administration. Some of the adverse effects are dizziness, confusion, headache, bradycardia, and diarrhea; however, these effects can be minimized by injecting the dosage over 20 minutes.[49] Ranitidine is contraindicated in patients having a history of a hypersensitivity to the drug or any of its components. With rapid injection of ranitidine in patients predisposed to cardiac rhythm disturbances, bradycardia can occur.[51]

Renal Imaging

Pharmacologic interventions during renal scintigraphy can be used to evaluate renovascular hypertension (RVH) or obstructive uropathy. The combination of radionuclide renography and angiotensin-converting enzyme (ACE) inhibition provides better identification of RVH than the use of radionuclide renography alone.[52] Pharmacologic interventions for radionuclidic evaluation of RVH use an ACE inhibitor either alone or in combination with furosemide. When furosemide is used with an ACE inhibitor, its purpose is to clear the renal collecting system of radioactivity in order to prevent interference with calculation of the cortical indices.[53] By itself, furosemide is used in renal scintigraphy to distinguish between dilatation of the collecting system resulting from mechanical obstruction and dilatation due to a distended and atonic but unobstructed collecting system.[54]

Captopril

Mechanism of Action

Captopril is an ACE inhibitor. ACE inhibitors block the conversion of angiotensin I to angiotensin II, decreasing angiotensin II-dependent postglomerular arteriole constriction and resulting in reduction of transcapillary forces maintaining glomerular filtration. Uptake of the pure glomerular filtration agent ^{99m}Tc-pentetate (^{99m}Tc-DTPA) in a kidney with renal artery stenosis tends to drop after ACE inhibition; however, there is no alteration in the unaffected kidney or kidneys of patients with essential hypertension. Uptake of ^{99m}Tc-mertiatide (^{99m}Tc-MAG3), a tubular agent, frequently remains unchanged after ACE inhibition unless severe stenosis is present. Cortical retention of ^{99m}Tc-MAG3 after ACE inhibition indicates RVH. A reduction in glomerular filtration as a result of ACE inhibition causes this cortical retention; the glomerular filtration decrease results in reduced urine flow in the renal tubules and delayed ^{99m}Tc-MAG3 washout. Cortical retention of ^{99m}Tc-DTPA can also result from decreased tubular flow.[52]

Dosage and Administration

With oral captopril, the patient should not eat any solids after midnight prior to the exam,[55] as food has been shown to decrease captopril absorption from the GI tract.[56] Hydration can be achieved by having the patient drink 7 mL/kg of water 30–60 minutes before the examination or by intravenously administering 10 mL/kg (maximum 500 mL) of 0.45% sodium chloride injection over 1 hour. During the study, an intravenous line should be open in case hypotension develops.[54] If two studies are conducted on the same day, continuing hydration between studies is recommended. Radiopharmaceutical administration occurs 60–90 minutes after oral ingestion of captopril so that peak blood levels of captopril can be achieved.[52] An acceptable dosage of captopril ranges from 25 mg to 50 mg, crushed and given orally with 150–250 mL of water. Unless the patient has poor absorption from the GI tract or delayed gastric emptying, a 25-mg dose is generally adequate.[57]

MTM Concerns

Since long-term use of ACE inhibitors may decrease the sensitivity of this test,[52] these medications should be withheld prior to the study according to their half-life. Short-acting ACE inhibitors should be discontinued for 2 or 3 days, and longer-acting products should be discontinued for 5–7 days. Withholding calcium-channel blockers and angiotensin-receptor blockers prior to the nuclear medicine study should also be considered. Diuretics should be discontinued prior to the exam in order to prevent dehydration.[54] It is important for the patient to be well hydrated upon arrival for the study.[55] When patients arrive relatively dehydrated, there is an increased risk of acute hypotension. Dehydration can also inhibit diuresis, leading to compromised interpretation of the exam by making it difficult to differentiate calyceal radioactivity resulting from dehydration and ACE inhibition-induced parenchymal retention.[52] Therefore, it is critical for the patient to drink water before arriving for the study to ensure adequate hydration.[55]

Before captopril administration, a baseline blood pressure must be obtained. During the study, blood pressure should monitored and recorded every 5–15 minutes.[52,54] If hypotension develops, the patient should be placed in a recumbent position, and if this is not sufficient to restore blood pressure, then normal saline should be infused. Establishment of an intravenous line prior to captopril administration is recommended in all high-risk patients, including those with a history of stroke, transient ischemic attacks, carotid disease, angina, and recent myocardial infarction. Patients should remain in the department until they are asymptomatic and standing blood pressure is at least 70% of baseline. Some centers require patient observation for an additional 30 minutes.[52]

Enalaprilat

Mechanism of Action

Enalaprilat, an ACE inhibitor that is administered intravenously, is a suitable alternative to captopril.[52] (See Mechanism of Action under Captopril, above.) Enalaprilat's hypotensive effect routinely occurs within 15 minutes of administration, and the maximal effect is seen at 1–4 hours.[52]

Dosage and Administration

The recommended intravenous dosage of enalaprilat is 40 μg/kg administered over 3–5 minutes, and the total dose should not exceed 2.5 mg.[58] (For recommendations regarding hydration and drugs to avoid prior to the study, see Dosage and Administration under Captopril.)

MTM Concerns

Before enalaprilat administration, a baseline blood pressure must be obtained. During the study, blood pressure should monitored and recorded every 5 minutes after enalaprilat administration.[52,54] An intravenous line for normal saline administration is recommended, since enalaprilat may increase the risk of hypotension.[52] (See MTM Concerns under Captopril.) It should be noted that enalaprilat has a longer duration of action than captopril.[58]

This intravenous agent reduces the procedure time and circumvents potential problems with poor absorption or delayed gastric emptying that can negatively affect the study when oral ACE inhibitors are used, but it does increase the potential for hypotension. Clinical studies indicate that RVH can be reliably identified when there is only a 10-minute delay between administration of enalaprilat and the radiopharmaceutical; however, the Consensus Report on ACEI Renography panel recommended a delay of 15 minutes between enalaprilat and radiopharmaceutical administration.[52]

Furosemide

Mechanism of Action

The diuretic action of furosemide is due to primary reabsorption of sodium and chloride in the proximal tubule, distal tubule, and loop of Henle. The drug's high degree of efficacy is due in large part to its unique site of action. The action on the distal tubule is not related to any inhibitory effect on aldosterone and carbonic anhydrase.[59] In normal patients, furosemide causes a strikingly increased flow of urine. When furosemide is given as an adjunct agent in nuclear medicine renography, there will be prompt washout of the radiopharmaceutical in a patient's dilated but nonobstructed collecting system.[54]

Dosage and Administration

The patient must be adequately hydrated prior to the study unless there is a contraindication to hydration.[58] The patient needs to maintain a urinary flow rate of 1–3 mL/minute during the examination. Upon arrival in the department, the patient should consume 500 mL of a beverage such as water or orange juice 15–30 minutes prior to the study. Some centers recommend that the patient's urine specific gravity be tested prior to the study and that the result be less than 1.015 to guarantee a reliable examination.[60] Some centers base the intravenous furosemide dose on creatinine levels, with doses ranging from 20 mg to 80 mg for adults,[54] while other centers recommend an adult intravenous dose of 40 mg.[60] For children, the intravenous dose of furosemide is 1 mg/kg for infants and 0.5 mg/kg for children 1–16 years of age.[60] The maximum recommended dose for children is 40 mg; however, some clinicians think a higher dose may be necessary in children with severe azotemia. Furosemide should be injected slowly over 1–2 minutes. A routinely used method is to inject furosemide 20 minutes after radiopharmaceutical administration. Other methods are also used, however; one method is to inject the radiopharmaceutical and furosemide at the same time, and another is to inject the furosemide 15 minutes before the radiopharmaceutical.[54]

MTM Concerns

Furosemide is contraindicated in patients with a history of hypersensitivity to furosemide and in those with anuria.[59] Patients who are dehydrated should not receive furosemide, because the resulting diuretic effect could compound the dehydration.[49] Some departments discontinue diuretics for 24 hours prior to the exam to reduce the possibility of dehydration.[55] Preexisting electrolyte depletion should be corrected before furosemide administration. Since electrolyte imbalance may occur when furosemide is given, the patient's electrolyte levels should be monitored.[61] Furosemide is a nonsulfonylarylamine sulfonamide,[8] and the package insert states that patients with an allergy to sulfonamides may also have an allergy to furosemide.[59] As discussed above under Acetazolamide MTM Concerns, the view of cross-reactivity between sulfonamides is controversial. Patients with a history of allergic reactions to drugs may have an elevated risk for all drug-induced adverse events that seem to be allergic in character.[9]

Because the maximal effect of furosemide occurs 15–18 minutes after intravenous administration, some centers administer it 15 minutes before the radiopharmaceutical. O'Reilly et al.[60] found no data supporting an increased dose of furosemide in azotemic patients. Damaged tubules respond poorly and slowly to any furosemide dose. Since the effect is slow and prolonged, furosemide does not induce the necessary acute stress to the obstructed segment.

Patients should be monitored for signs of hypotension after furosemide administration. Other potential adverse effects are nausea, vomiting, diarrhea, dizziness, headache, tinnitus, rash, electrolyte depletion, and dehydration.[49]

Conclusion

Pharmacologic interventional agents play a significant role in nuclear medicine procedures. Thus, it is critical for the health care professional to be aware of contraindications and precautions concerning these pharmaceuticals as well as the treatment of adverse events. Although not all inclusive, this chapter covers the interventional agents most frequently used in nuclear medicine studies.

References

1. Mettler FA Jr, Guiberteau MJ. Cerebrovascular system. In: Mettler FA Jr, Guiberteau MJ, eds. *Essentials of Nuclear Medicine Imaging.* 5th ed. Philadelphia: Saunders Elsevier; 2006:53–73.
2. Sterile Acetazolamide Sodium, USP [package insert]. Bedford, OH: Bedford Laboratories; 1995.
3. Ziessman HA, O'Malley JP, Thrall JH. Central nervous system. In: Thrall JH, ed. *Nuclear Medicine: The Requisites in Radiology.* 3rd ed. Philadelphia: Elsevier Mosby; 2006:419–49.
4. Asenbaum S, Reinprecht A, Brücke T, et al. A study of acetazolamide-induced changes in cerebral blood flow using ^{99m}Tc HMPAO SPECT in patients with cerebrovascular disease. *Neuroradiology.* 1995;37:13–9.
5. Shackett P. Brain SPECT. In: McGrew L, ed. *Nuclear Medicine Technology Procedures and Quick Reference.* Philadelphia: Lippincott Williams & Wilkins; 2000:40–5.

6. Yudd AP, Van Heertum RL, Masdeu JC. Interventions and functional brain imaging. *Semin Nucl Med.* 1991;21:153–8.
7. Acetazolamide Drugdex evaluations. Micromedex. www.thomsonhc.com. Accessed May 18, 2010 (access available only to subscribers).
8. Johnson KK, Green DL, Rife JP, et al. Sulfonamide cross-reactivity: fact or fiction? *Ann Pharmacother.* 2005;39:290–301.
9. Strom BL, Schinnar R, Apter AJ, et al. Absence of cross-reactivity between sulfonamide antibiotics and sulfonamide nonantibiotics. *N Engl J Med.* 2003;349:1628–35.
10. DePuey EG, Rozanski A. Pharmacological and other nonexercise alternatives to exercise testing to evaluate myocardial perfusion and left ventricular function with radionuclides. *Semin Nucl Med.* 1991;21:92–101.
11. Strauss HW, Miller DD, Wittry MD, et al. Procedure guideline for myocardial perfusion imaging 3. 3. *J Nucl Med Technol.* 2008;36:155–61.
12. Crawford ES, Husain SS. Pharmacologic stress. In: Crawford ES, ed. *Nuclear Cardiac Imaging Terminology and Technical Aspects.* Reston, VA: Society of Nuclear Medicine; 2003:16–25.
13. Ziessman HA, O'Malley JP, Thrall JH. Cardiac system. In: Thrall JH, ed. *Nuclear Medicine: The Requisites in Radiology.* 3rd ed. Philadelphia: Elsevier Mosby; 2006: 450–507.
14. Adenoscan [package insert]. Deerfield, IL: Astellas Pharma US; 2005.
15. Mettler FA Jr, Guiberteau MJ. Cardiovascular system. In: Mettler FA Jr, Guiberteau MJ, eds. *Essentials of Nuclear Medicine Imaging.* 5th ed. Philadelphia: Saunders Elsevier; 2006:101–57.
16. Bokhari S, Ficaro EP, McCallister BD. Adenosine stress protocols for myocardial perfusion imaging. *J Nucl Cardiol.* 2007;14:415–6.
17. Druz RS. Current advances in vasodilator pharmacological stress perfusion imaging. *Semin Nucl Med.* 2009;39:204–9.
18. Leppo JA. Dipyridamole myocardial perfusion imaging. *J Nucl Med.* 1994;35:730–3.
19. Dipyridamole Injection USP [package insert]. Bedford, OH: Bedford Laboratories; 2007.
20. I.V. Persantine product monograph. Billerica, MA: Du Pont Merck; 1990.
21. Verani MS, Mahmarian JJ. Pharmacological stress nuclear cardiology imaging. *Am J Card Imaging.* 1994;8:223–30.
22. Botvinick EH. Current methods of pharmacologic stress testing and the potential advantages of new agents. *J Nucl Med Technol.* 2009;37:14–25.
23. Kowalsky RJ, Falen SW. Heart. In: Kowalsky RJ, Falen SW, eds. *Radiopharmaceuticals in Nuclear Pharmacy and Nuclear Medicine.* 2nd ed. Washington, DC: American Pharmacists Association; 2004:515–60.
24. Miyamoto MI, Vemotico SL, Majmundar H, et al. Pharmacologic stress myocardial perfusion imaging: a practical approach. *J Nucl Cardiol.* 2007;14:250–5.
25. Lexiscan [package insert]. Deerfield, IL: Astellas Pharma US; 2009.
26. Swanson DP. Radiopharmaceuticals for endocrine imaging: adrenocortical imaging. In: Swanson DP, Chilton HM, Thrall JH, eds. *Pharmaceuticals in Medical Imaging: Radiopaque Contrast Media, Radiopharmaceuticals, Enhancement Agents for Magnetic Resonance Imaging and Ultrasound.* New York: Macmillan; 1990:360–8.
27. Ziessman HA, O'Malley JP, Thrall JH. Endocrine system. In: Thrall JH, ed. *Nuclear Medicine: The Requisites in Radiology.* 3rd ed. Philadelphia: Elsevier Mosby; 2006: 71–112.

28. Dexamethasone Drugdex evaluations. Micromedex. www.thomsonhc.com. Accessed August 25, 2010 (access available only to subscribers).
29. Swanson DP, Dick TJ. Appendix C: Drugs for the mitigation of internal radiocontamination. In: Swanson DP, Chilton HM, Thrall JH, eds. *Pharmaceuticals in Medical Imaging: Radiopaque Contrast Media, Radiopharmaceuticals, Enhancement Agents for Magnetic Resonance Imaging and Ultrasound.* New York: Macmillan; 1990:690–707.
30. AdreView [package insert]. Arlington Heights, IL: GE Healthcare; 2008.
31. Kowalsky RJ, Falen SW. Thyroid. In: Kowalsky RJ, Falen SW, eds. *Radiopharmaceuticals in Nuclear Pharmacy and Nuclear Medicine.* 2nd ed. Washington, DC: American Pharmacists Association; 2004:495–513.
32. Iodine Drugdex evaluations. Micromedex. www.thomsonhc.com. Accessed May 8, 2010 (access available only to subscribers).
33. Unclassified therapeutic agents: potassium perchlorate. In: *AHFS Drug Information.* Bethesda, MD: American Society of Health-System Pharmacists; 1996:2767–8.
34. Potassium perchlorate Drugdex evaluations. Micromedex. www.thomsonhc.com. Accessed May 8, 2010 (access available only to subscribers).
35. Chen M-K, Doddamane I, Cheng DW. Recombinant human thyroid-stimulating hormone as an alternative for thyroid hormone withdrawal in thyroid cancer management. *Curr Opin Oncol.* 2010;22:6–10.
36. Thyrotropin Drugdex evaluations. Micromedex. www.thomsonhc.com. Accessed August 27, 2010 (access available only to subscribers).
37. Thyrogen thyrotropin alfa for injection [package insert]. Cambridge, MA: Genzyme Corporation; 2004.
38. Ziessman HA, O'Malley JP, Thrall JH. Hepatobiliary system. In: Thrall JH, ed. *Nuclear Medicine: The Requisites in Radiology.* 3rd ed. Philadelphia: Elsevier Mosby; 2006:159–214.
39. Sargent EN, Meyers HI, Hubsher J. Cholecystokinetic cholecystography: efficacy and tolerance study of sincalide. *AJR Am J Roentgenol.* 1976;127:267–71.
40. Ziessman HA. Nuclear medicine hepatobiliary imaging. *Clin Gastroenterol Hepatol.* 2010;8:111–6.
41. Kinevac [package insert]. Bedford, OH: Ben Venue Laboratories (Manufactured for Bracco Diagnostics, Princeton NJ); 2008.
42. Shackett P. HIDA. In: McGrew L, ed. *Nuclear Medicine Technology Procedures and Quick Reference.* Philadelphia: Lippincott Williams & Wilkins; 2000:134–40.
43. Fink-Bennett D. Augmented cholescintigraphy: its role in detecting acute and chronic disorders of the hepatobiliary tree. *Semin Nucl Med.* 1991;21:128–39.
44. Mettler FA Jr, Guiberteau MJ. Gastrointestinal tract. In: Mettler FA Jr, Guiberteau MJ, eds. *Essentials of Nuclear Medicine Imaging.* 5th ed. Philadelphia: Saunders Elsevier; 2006:203–42.
45. Chilton HM, Brown ML. Radiopharmaceuticals for abdominal and gastrointestinal imaging: reticuloendothelial, hepatobiliary, and intestinal. In: Swanson DP, Chilton HM, Thrall JH, eds. *Pharmaceuticals in Medical Imaging: Radiopaque Contrast Media, Radiopharmaceuticals, Enhancement Agents for Magnetic Resonance Imaging and Ultrasound.* New York: Macmillan; 1990:462–500.
46. Ziessman HA, O'Malley JP, Thrall JH. Gastrointestinal system. In: Thrall JH, ed. *Nuclear Medicine: The Requisites in Radiology.* 3rd ed. Philadelphia: Elsevier Mosby; 2006:346–83.
47. Ford PV, Bartold SP, Fink-Bennett DM, et al. Procedure guideline for gastrointestinal bleeding and Meckel's diverticulum scintigraphy. *J Nucl Med.* 1999;40:1226–32.

48. Shackett P. Meckel's diverticulum. In: McGrew L, ed. *Nuclear Medicine Technology Procedures and Quick Reference.* Philadelphia, PA: Lippincott Williams & Wilkins; 2000:178–82.
49. Park H-M, Duncan K. Nonradioactive pharmaceuticals in nuclear medicine. *J Nucl Med Technol.* 1994;22:240–9.
50. Cimetidine Drugdex evaluations. Micromedex. www.thomsonhc.com. Accessed August 27, 2010 (access available only to subscribers).
51. Ranitidine Drugdex evaluations. Micromedex. www.thomsonhc.com. Accessed August 27, 2010 (access available only to subscribers).
52. Taylor A, Nally J, Aurell M, et al. Consensus report on ACE inhibitor renography for detecting renovascular hypertension. In: Taylor A, Nally JV, Thomsen H, eds. *Radionuclides in Nephrourology.* Reston, VA: Society of Nuclear Medicine; 1997:8–21.
53. Mettler FA Jr, Guiberteau MJ. Genitourinary system and adrenal glands. In: Mettler FA Jr, Guiberteau MJ, eds. *Essentials of Nuclear Medicine Imaging.* 5th ed. Philadelphia: Saunders Elsevier; 2006:293–324.
54. Ziessman HA, O'Malley JP, Thrall JH. Genitourinary system. In: Thrall JH, ed. *Nuclear Medicine: The Requisites in Radiology.* 3rd ed. Philadelphia: Elsevier Mosby; 2006:215–62.
55. Taylor A, Schuster DM, Alazraki N. Genitourinary system. In: Taylor A, Schuster DM, Alazraki N, eds. *A Clinician's Guide to Nuclear Medicine.* 2nd ed. Reston, VA: Society of Nuclear Medicine; 2006:45–74.
56. Captopril Drugdex evaluations. Micromedex. www.thomsonhc.com. Accessed August 20, 2010 (access available only to subscribers).
57. Fine EJ. Interventions in renal scintirenography. *Semin Nucl Med.* 1991;21:116–27.
58. Sfakianakis GN, Georgiou M, Cavagnaro F, et al. Fast protocols for obstruction (diuretic renography) and for renovascular hypertension (ACE inhibition). *J Nucl Med Technol.* 1992;20:193–206.
59. Furosemide Injection, USP 10 mg/mL [package insert]. Shirley, NY: American Regent Laboratories; 1997.
60. O'Reilly P, Aurell M, Britton K, et al. Consensus on diuresis renography for investigating the dilated upper urinary tract. In: Taylor A, Nally JV, Thomsen H, eds. *Radionuclides in Nephrourology.* Reston, VA: Society of Nuclear Medicine; 1997:1–7.
61. Furosemide Drugdex evaluations. Micromedex. www.thomsonhc.com. Accessed August 26, 2010 (access available only to subscribers).

CHAPTER 9

Review of Imaging Procedures Using Magnetic Resonance Imaging

Sam Baird, Dee H. Wu, and Blaine Templar Smith

Pharmacists have an increasing role in the use of contrast agents in imaging. In 2008 a representative of the Joint Commission, which accredits health care facilities, discussed that growing role for pharmacists in contrast agent use during a meeting of the American Society of Health-System Pharmacists.[1] The Joint Commission's goal is to "improve health care for the public, in collaboration with other stakeholders, by evaluating health care organizations and inspiring them to excel in providing safe and effective care of the highest quality and value."[2] Since pharmacists will likely have greater oversight of and accountability for contrast agents, they may be given additional responsibilities such as verifying contrast agent doses, reviewing the storage of contrast agents, and verifying the indications for use.[1]

It is likely that health-system pharmacists will become part of the team providing magnetic resonance (MR) imaging. Typically, a radiologist acts as the overseer of the imaging process. Others on the team include MR technologists, medical physicists, MR vendor service personnel, and hospital administrators. One of the radiologist's responsibilities is assessing the appropriateness of requested MR examinations, including the appropriate use of gadolinium, a contrast agent used in some MR procedures to enhance images (see Chapter 10).

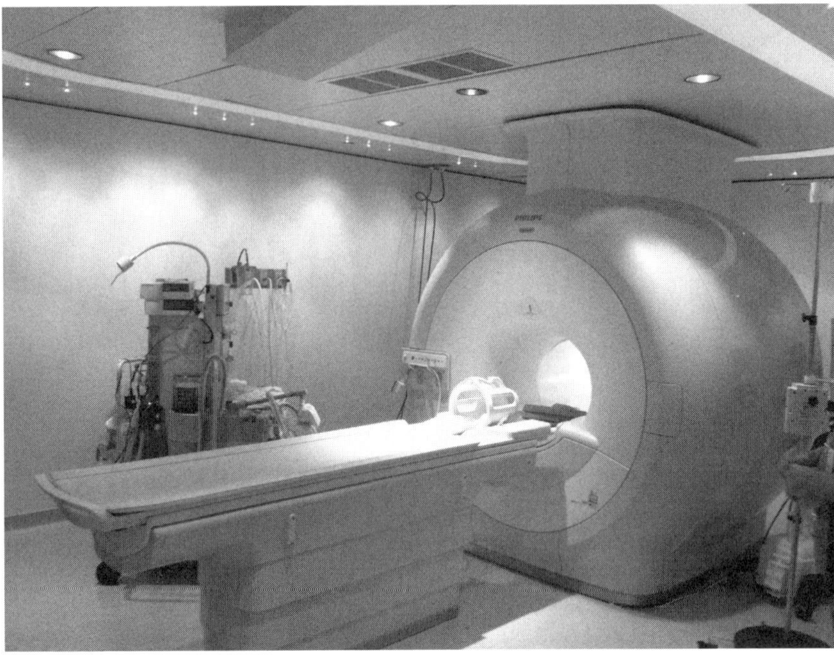

Figure 9-1. Equipment for magnetic resonance imaging (MRI).

In MR imaging, the patient typically lies on a movable table. The movable table slowly carries the patient through the apparatus (Figure 9-1), which is composed of a scanner and several coils. The coils produce varying magnetic fields; this is the means by which MR scanning is produced, using radio signals to create cross-sectional images of the area of interest or of the whole patient.

Clinical Role of MRI

Magnetic resonance imaging (MRI) helps improve visualization of pathology. Most disease states, including tumors (benign or malignant) are accompanied by some degree of edema (accumulation of excess intercellular fluid). The edema fluid is mostly water but may include proteins, carbohydrates, and fats, depending on the pathologic process. Often, it is the edema that helps distinguish pathologic from normal tissues. MRI is very sensitive to the presence and extent of water in soft tissues. A comparison of a noncontrast x-ray computed tomography (CT) image of a brain (Figure 9-2) and the more definitive MR image (Figure 9-3) illustrates the advantage of MRI.

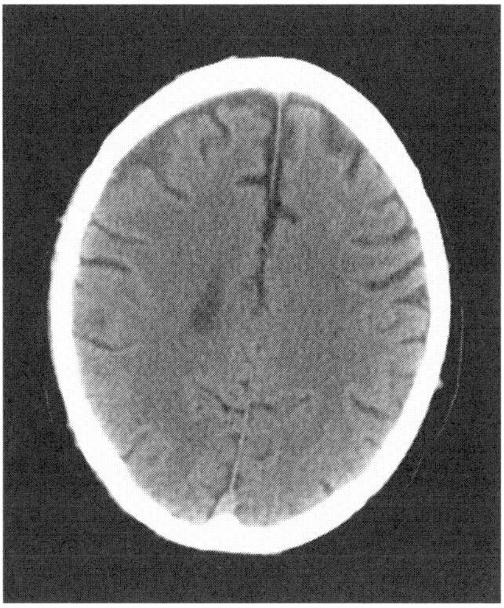

Figure 9-2. Noncontrast x-ray computed tomography (CT) brain image.

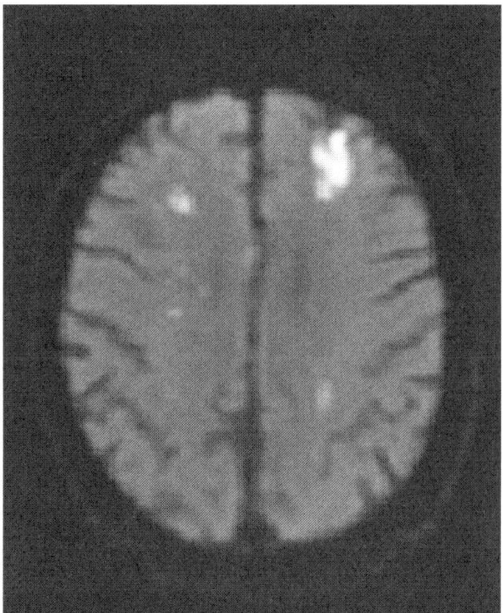

Figure 9-3. Magnetic resonance imaging (MRI) brain image (diffusion-weighted).

Figure 9-3 shows a *diffusion-weighted* image. It clearly reveals multiple small, scattered infarcts (the white lesions). Diffusion-weighted images are manipulated to show areas that have unusual diffusion as bright spots. The bright spots indicate areas of increased (water) diffusion, and damage. An infarct in its early stages is characterized by an increase in edema (i.e., water) and would not be visible in a CT image (Figure 9-2, obtained shortly before Figure 9-3).

In addition to edema, pathology is frequently accompanied by increased vascularity (e.g., vascular abnormalities such as aneurysms and arteriovenous malformations, tumors, infectious and inflammatory processes). MRI capitalizes on this increased vascularity by using gadolinium as an intravenous contrast agent to reveal more distinctly the areas of increased vascularity. Often, a pathologic process sequesters more contrast agent than do nonpathologic tissues, increasing the visibility of the pathologic tissue. Thus, through separate mechanisms, edema and contrast agents highlight pathology.

In many circumstances, MRI without contrast can be used. Noncontrast MRI can be used to observe the movement of liquids such as blood and cerebrospinal fluid. The imaging of arterial blood flow is termed *MR angiography (MRA).*

MRI Hardware

The three major instruments needed to create an image are the main magnet, the radiofrequency (RF) pulse generator, and the gradient coils (typically three, an x, y, and z coil). The main magnet is the central field which, in turn, creates the electromagnetic environment for magnetic resonance. This hardware is used to create signals from the hydrogen atoms in the patient's soft tissues, through the application of an electromagnetic field. This is why the presence of water is key: water contains hydrogen atoms.

MRI Signal Creation

The basis of MRI is the hydrogen atom, primarily as it is bound in the water molecule. Approximately 60% of the human body weight and approximately 98% to 99% of the molecules in the human body are composed of water. There are approximately 4.7×10^{28} hydrogen atoms in the body, compared with approximately 1.4×10^{28} oxygen atoms and 4.2×10^{27} carbon atoms in the body.[3] It is this overwhelming abundance of hydrogen atoms that makes MRI possible. Although other atoms can be used for MRI, their use is impractical because of their relative paucity in the body.

The hydrogen atom consists of one proton. Unlike other atoms, the hydrogen atom does not have an electron (except in its ground state, which is not pertinent to MRI). Therefore, in this chapter the terms *hydrogen atom, hydrogen proton,* and *proton* will be used interchangeably.

The hydrogen proton is constantly spinning (termed *precession* in MRI nomenclature); that is, it rotates in a 360° circle like a toy top. Like a top, the hydrogen atom also spins at an angle to its longitudinal axis (Figure 9-4). The spinning of the proton results in a positive electric charge that is accompanied by a magnetic field. Every magnetic field has a vector and has direction. This electromagnetic field (B_0) created by the spinning hydrogen proton, possessing vector and direction, is the foundation of MRI (Figure 9-5).

When the patient lies in the external magnet, the parallel vector of each hydrogen proton adds up to a cumulative vector superimposed upon the vector of the external magnet. This magnetization of the patient's hydrogen protons caused by the external magnet is called *longitudinal magnetization.*

When the RF pulse is turned on and absorbed by the patient's hydrogen protons, the magnetic field or vector of the patient, caused by the patient's hydrogen protons, is deflected or "tipped" transverse to the magnetic field of the external magnet (Figure 9-6). This new direction of magnetization is referred to as "tipped" magnetization in the transverse plane. Depending on the strength and duration of the RF pulse, the magnetic vector of the hydrogen protons in the patient's body

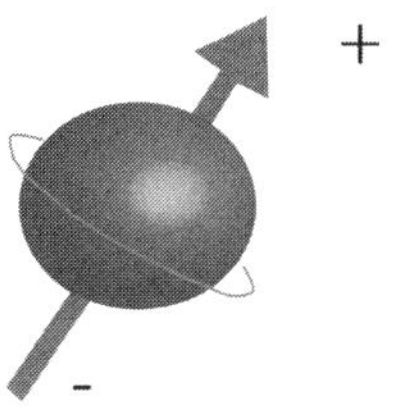

Figure 9-4. Each hydrogen atom (proton) has an electric charge that is constantly spinning. Another way to visualize the magnetic dipole is as an electric charge revolving around an infinitesimal area. The electric charge and spinning create a magnetic field. Each proton then has a small electromagnetic field and acts as a small bar magnet. Obeying Faraday's law, a small changing electric field results in a small magnetic field.

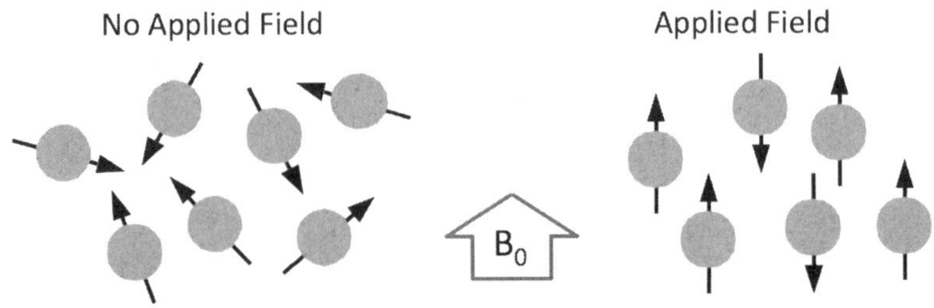

Figure 9-5. Normally, protons are aligned in a random manner (left). This changes (right) when they are exposed to a strong external magnetic field (B_0). Then they are aligned in only one of two ways, either parallel or antiparallel to the external magnetic field. A slightly larger portion of protons is aligned parallel to the magnetic field than antiparallel to the magnetic field. For every 10 million antiparallel protons there are approximately 10,000,007 parallel protons—a very slight, but usable, difference.

can be tipped from 0° to 180° transverse to the main vector of the external magnet. The "tipping" of the patient's magnetic vector is crucial for the generation and measurement of the MRI signal (Figure 9-7).

Relaxation and the T1 and T2 Concepts

Basic to making the MR signal that is needed to create an image is the phenomenon of relaxation. As used here, the term *relaxation* describes the time-varying changes associated with the discharge and exchange of magnetic energy from and within ensembles of hydrogen protons.[4] The hydrogen protons are said to "relax" to their preexisting steady

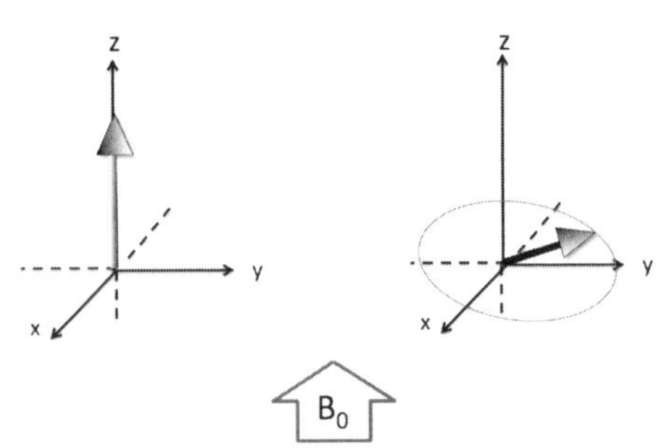

Figure 9-6. Using the 90° radiofrequency (RF) pulse to tip the magnetization vector, magnetization changes from the longitudinal plane (left) to the transverse plane (right).

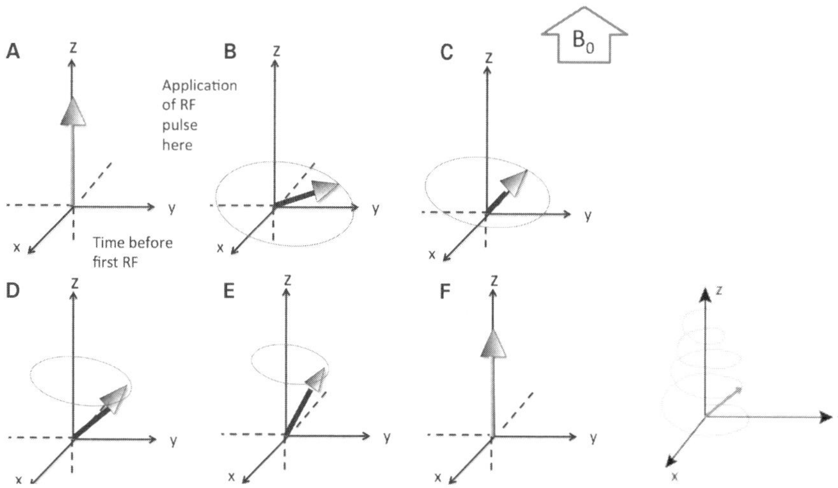

Figure 9-7. Before the RF pulse (A) there is only longitudinal magnetization. Immediately after the 90° RF pulse there is no longitudinal magnetization. Instead, there is new transverse magnetization. The RF pulse "tips" the patient's magnetic field from the longitudinal plane into the transverse plane (B, and illustration on right), and this transverse magnetization vector is spinning around. With time, the tipped protons relax to their original positions (C, D, E, F).

state parallel to the main magnetic field as they exchange the energy absorbed from the RF pulse (Figure 9-7 C, D, E, F). It is this discharged energy that the receiver in the MR hardware "hears" and converts to make the MR image. The two principal relaxation processes are termed *T1* or *spin-lattice* relaxation and *T2* or *spin-spin* relaxation, respectively (further described below). T1, or spin-lattice, relaxation results in T1 contrast. T2, or spin-spin, relaxation results in T2 contrast.[5] T1 relaxation and T2 relaxation account for the exquisite contrast often seen within soft tissues on MRI (Figure 9-8).

By manipulating imaging techniques to extract contrast attributable to T1 and T2 differences, it is possible to accentuate different soft tissues and increase the visibility of pathology they may harbor. As noted, some degree of edema accompanies most disease states, and edema is mostly water. Many tumors, benign or malignant, have increased water content, distinguishing them from normal tissue. The T2-weighted pulse sequences (in which the signal is manipulated to return in a delayed fashion) are very sensitive to water and are invaluable

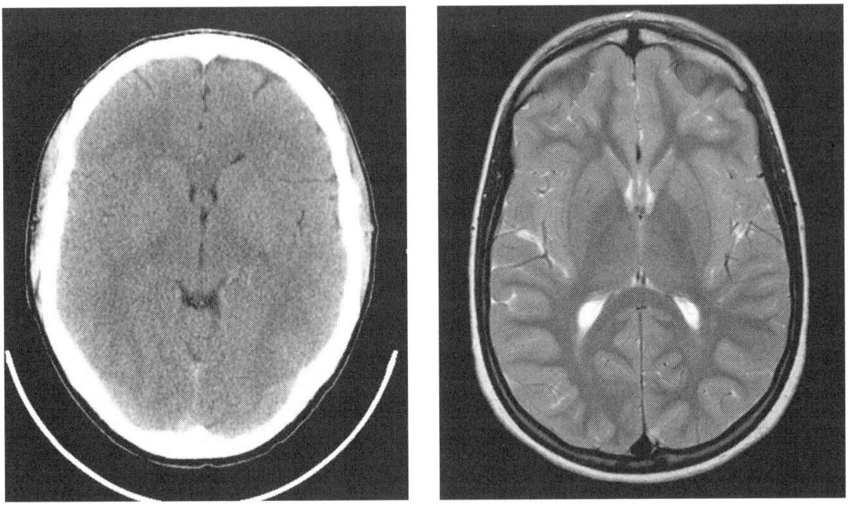

Figure 9-8. Comparison of MRI (right) and CT (left). There is more contrast and greater ease of identification of the different parts of the brain in the MRI sample. The increased contrast between different soft tissues in the brain is due to their differing T1 and T2 relaxation characteristics.

in the detection of pathologic edema. MRI without the use of a contrast agent may be thought of as imaging the increased water in pathologic tissues. Manipulation of the T1 and T2 differences between different soft tissues discharging their energy from the RF pulse allows unlimited imaging strategies to create differences in contrast between the different soft tissues. This ability to exploit T1 and T2 differences gives MRI a considerable advantage over CT in the differentiation of soft tissues. Often, different soft tissues that appear on CT to blend together are readily distinguishable on MRI, usually without intravenous contrast.

T1 Relaxation (Spin-Lattice Relaxation)

In T1 or spin-lattice relaxation, the hydrogen atom discharges a portion of the energy to its immediate surroundings (i.e., its lattice or neighborhood). An analogy would be the melting of ice. When ice melts, it exchanges its energy with the adjacent atmosphere (environment or lattice), going from a solid (ice) to a liquid (water). The lattice can be thought of as the environment of adjacent soft tissues that directly interplay with the hydrogen protons discharging their recently acquired RF energy. The hydrogen protons discharge this energy so they can return to the longitudinal equilibrium state. As the hydrogen atoms discharge their energy, they begin to realign with the magnetic field of the external magnet, and there is progressive loss of transverse magnetization and progressive rebuilding of longitudinal magnetization. Because of their different chemical compositions, different tissues in the body discharge the energy from their hydrogen atoms at different rates. For example, fat discharges its energy from the RF pulse much faster than does free water (e.g., cerebrospinal fluid). It is this difference in the time of discharging energy that allows the creation of tissue contrast in MRI.

T2 Relaxation (Spin-Spin Relaxation)

When the protons are aligned with the main field of the external magnet (longitudinal magnetization), they are all precessing (spinning at the same speed) at their normal frequency. However, the protons are not in phase with each other. To use the analogy of a clock face,[6] each proton circles the clock face every 12 hours. If the protons are not in phase with each other, each proton points to a different location on the clock face. If each proton points to the same location on the clock face, they are in phase with each other. The RF pulse not only tips the protons' magnetic vector transverse to the field of the external magnet but also puts the protons in phase with each other, making them synchronous with each other, or giving them *phase coherence* (the same, or uniform, phase). Consider an example involving five wristwatches. Each watch is on a 12-hour cycle (or frequency). However, each watch is set at a different time (e.g., 1 o'clock, 4 o'clock). If each watch on the 12-hour cycle is at the same time (e.g., 2 o'clock), they are in phase with each other; that is, they are synchronized. The RF pulse puts the precessing protons into phase with one another. However, as soon as the RF pulse is turned off, the protons begin to lose phase (i.e., phase coherence) with one another. As the protons lose phase with each other, there is a corresponding loss of transverse magnetization. The loss of magnetization in the transverse plane is termed T2 relaxation, or spin-spin relaxation.

MRI Procedure

The MR signal is created by (1) energy released from T1 relaxation (as the proton regains its longitudinal alignment with the vector of the magnet) combined with (2) energy released from T2 relaxation as the proton loses phase coherency in the transverse plane. The signal for the MR image is created in the following manner. A 90° RF pulse is sent into the magnet. After the 90° RF pulse, at a predetermined time, a 180° RF pulse is sent into the magnet. Next, after a predetermined time (the readout time), the radio receiver listens for and records the signal originating from the relaxing protons. The signal recorded by the receiver is termed the *echo,* because it is the echo of the protons at the time of the 180° RF pulse. The time from the 90° pulse to the echo is termed *TE* (time to echo), or *echo time* (Figure 9-9). To create one image, this pulse sequence may be repeated several times. This repetition allows for averaging of the signals to obtain the best image. The time between repetition of the 90° RF pulse is known as *TR* (time to repetition), or *repetition time.* An example of how T1 and T2 are used is shown in Figure 9-10.

Fluid-attenuated inversion recovery (FLAIR) is a method used to suppress the signal from fluids and emphasize tissues. Other methods of manipulating the signal and return echo are used to enhance particular types of images. These include *STIR* and *diffusion-weighted* sequences. STIR stands for short T1 inversion recovery; it is a particular pulse sequence designed to suppress the signal from fat. A diffusion-weighted setting is designed to emphasize small changes in water movement

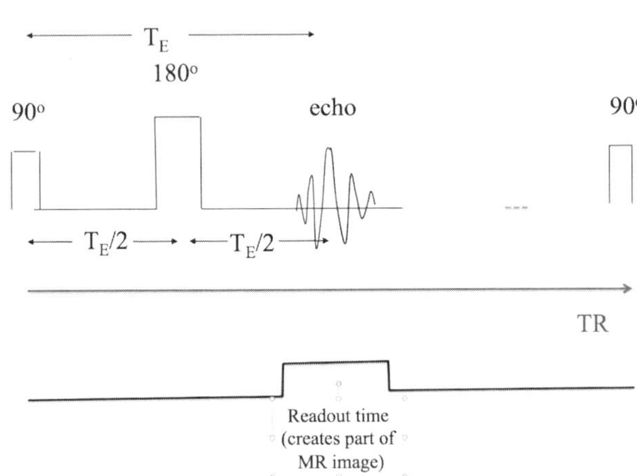

Figure 9-9. Schematic for the traditional T2 spin echo pulse sequence. The 90° radiofrequency (RF) pulse is the start of the race, the 180° RF pulse is the "turn around" command and the echo, i.e., when the radio receiver hears (the readout time), and the rephased T2 signal is when the runners return to the starting line.

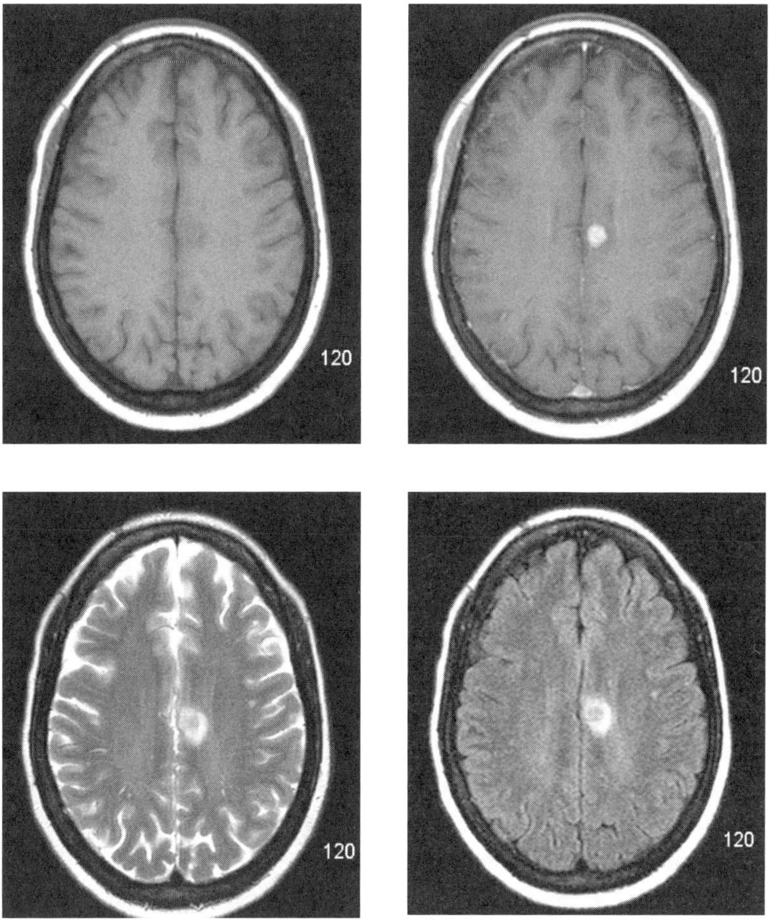

Figure 9-10. Top: T1 sequence without contrast (left) and T1 sequence with contrast (right). Bottom: T2 pulse sequence (left) and FLAIR pulse sequence (right). The abnormality (a metastasis) is barely visible in the no-contrast T1 image (top left). With contrast (intravenous gadolinium), the lesion is readily apparent (top right). The T2 and FLAIR images (bottom) reveal the edema around the lesion, further characterizing the lesion.

(areas of restricted diffusion) inside injured areas. Differing pathologies may be more apparent on one pulse sequence than on another pulse sequence. The T1 with contrast, T2, FLAIR, STIR, and diffusion-weighted sequences are just a few of the pulse sequences that have been developed to exploit the T1 and T2 differences among soft tissues and between pathologic and nonpathologic tissues on MRI.

Use of Gradients to Localize the Signal

The task of sequentially imaging succeeding portions of the patient's body (slice image location) is accomplished by the application of three gradients to the main magnet. With the superimposed gradients, the strength of the external magnet is weaker at the patient's feet and becomes progressively stronger as it moves toward the patient's head. This difference allows for localization of the MR signal from different parts of the body into a two-dimensional image. By using three gradients in the x, y, and z planes, the origin of any signal from the patient can be plotted into a representational composite picture.

Conclusion

As their roles and responsibilities grow within clinical environments, pharmacists will be working more directly with radiologists and other diagnostic imaging staff to establish procedures that follow the indications and routines for improved safety and best practices in patient care. This chapter provides a general description of how MRI works and the clinical importance of MRI.

References

1. Rich DS. The Joint Commission perspective on contrast agents: requirements and tips for success. 2008. http://esymposia.ashp.org/collaboration/overview.htm. Accessed February 8, 2010.
2. The Joint Commission. Mission. www.jointcommission.org/. Accessed August 11, 2011.
3. Thomas Jefferson National Accelerator Facility. How many atoms are in the human body? http://education.jlab.org/qa/mathatom_04.html. Accessed 2010.
4. Brown MA, Semelka RC. *MRI: Basic Principles and Applications.* 4th ed. Hoboken, NJ: Wiley-Blackwell; 2010.
5. Bushberg J, Seibert JA, Leidholdt EM Jr, et al. *The Essential Physics of Medical Imaging.* 2nd ed. New York: Lippincott Williams & Wilkins; 2001:933.
6. Westbrook C, Roth CK, Talbot J. *MRI in Practice.* New York: Wiley-Blackwell; 2005.

CHAPTER 10

Adjunct Agents Used in Magnetic Resonance Imaging

Contrast Media

Vivian S. Loveless

The use of paramagnetic metal ions to assist in acquiring magnetic resonance (MR) data began with the phenomenal discovery of nuclear magnetic resonance. In 1978, the use of paramagnetic ions was first demonstrated in tissue when a manganese compound was injected into dogs with myocardial infarctions and the researchers discovered not only differential uptake of manganese by infarcted and normal tissue but also different tissue relaxation rates. In the 1980s, gadolinium diethylenetriamine pentaacetate (Gd-DTPA) was the first paramagnetic chelate approved for clinical use in humans.[1]

Contrast Role in Imaging

MR imaging contrast agents used clinically are heavy metal chelates; they are classified as either paramagnetic or superparamagnetic contrast agents.[2,3] To be safe and effective, these contrast media have two primary requirements: that the compound be biocompatible, and that the agent adequately enhance the relaxation rate of tissue-water protons. The factors dictating contrast agents' biocompatibility are pharmacokinetics, biodistribution, stability, and toxicity.[1] Binding the heavy metal to a ligand in a chelate minimizes the inherent toxicity associated with the heavy metal.[3]

These contrast agents decrease the longitudinal (spin-lattice) relaxation time (T1) as well as the transverse (spin-spin) relaxation time (T2) of water protons in close proximity. The use of paramagnetic or superparamagnetic contrast agents with MR imaging yields an enhanced image.[2] This image enhancement is due to the ability of the MR contrast agents to change the tissue relaxation times and thus manipulate the tissue signal intensity on MR imaging.[4]

Paramagnetic Contrast Agents: Gadolinium Agents

The active constituents of the paramagnetic MR imaging contrast agents approved for use and available in the United States are gadolinium ions. Gadolinium diethylenetriamine pentaacetic acid (Gd-DTPA), also known as gadopentetate dimeglumine, was the first MRI contrast agent to receive approval for use in the United States.[4] There are two categories of gadolinium contrast agents: nonspecific extracellular gadolinium chelates and high-relaxivity contrast agents. With both types of compounds, the gadolinium heavy metal is bound to a ligand. These contrast agents also are categorized according to the chemical structure of the ligand, which can be either linear or cyclic and may be ionic or nonionic. The ionic compounds exhibit a charge in solution. Kinetic, thermodynamic, and conditional stability factors determine the stability of gadolinium contrast agents. Gadolinium contrast agents with cyclic ligands have greater stability than agents with linear ligands.[3] Gadolinium contrast agents are called positive contrast agents, since the signal on T1-weighted images tends to appear brighter than the surrounding tissues.[3,5]

Dosage and Administration of Nonspecific Gadolinium Agents

The nonspecific gadolinium chelates are dosed on a millimole per kilogram or, often, a milliliter per kilogram basis. Their administration is either by rapid intravenous (IV) infusion or by IV bolus injection,[6] and their biodistribution and pharmacokinetics mimic those of radiographic iodine-based contrast media.[3,7] The four classes of nonspecific extracellular gadolinium chelates are (1) nonionic, linear ligand;

(2) ionic, linear ligand; (3) nonionic, cyclic ligand; and (4) ionic, cyclic ligand.[3] Table 10-1 gives examples of the four classes of nonspecific extracellular gadolinium chelates, including the agents currently available in the United States, along with the package insert recommended dosages.

Nonspecific extracellular gadolinium chelates are hydrophilic complexes that do not cross the intact blood–brain barrier.[12] After IV injection, these agents are not protein bound and they undergo renal excretion[3] via glomerular filtration.[12] In vivo biotransformation or decomposition has not been detected, and more than 95% of the administered agent is excreted in the urine in the first 24 hours after injection.[12]

Dosage and Administration of High-Relaxivity Gadolinium Agents

The high-relaxivity agents are water-soluble agents[13,14] with ionic, linear ligands.[3] These agents do not cross the blood–brain barrier[13,14] and, in general, they behave similarly to the nonspecific extracellular agents immediately after intravascular administration. However, in contrast to the nonspecific extracellular gadolinium chelates, two of the high-relaxivity agents, gadofosveset and gadoxetate, are protein bound and undergo some degree of biliary excretion.[3]

Gadofosveset trisodium exhibits 79.8% to 87.4% protein binding, which results in longer vascular residence time and enhances the MR relaxivity of the gadolinium complex. This agent is approved in the United States for magnetic resonance angiography (MRA) because of the increased residence time in the blood. Gadofosveset is excreted by slow renal elimination; 83.5% is eliminated in the urine over 14 days, with most of the renal excretion occurring in the first 72 hours.[15] Approximately 4.7% of the gadofosveset dose is eliminated via the feces.[16]

Gadoxetate disodium is a hydrophilic, highly water-soluble compound, but it also contains a lipophilic moiety. It demonstrates weak (less than 10%), transient protein binding,[13] and elimination is equal between the renal and hepatobiliary routes.[13,17] Because of the biliary excretion, the high-relaxivity agent gadoxetate can be used as an adjunct in liver imaging.[3]

The third high-relaxivity agent, gadobenate dimeglumine, is primarily used as an extracellular agent.[3] This agent exhibits low, weak, and transient plasma protein binding but does not undergo metabolism,

Table 10-1. Nonspecific Extracellular Gadolinium Chelates[3,6,8–11]

Class of Ligands	Examples	Dosage
Nonionic, linear	Gadoversetamide (Optimark [Covidien]) 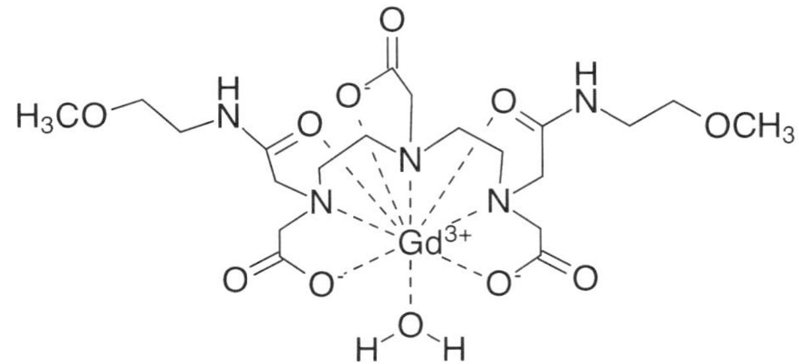	*Central nervous system (CNS) and Liver:* 0.2 mL/kg (0.1 mmol/kg) as bolus IV injection at 1–2 mL/second *Pediatrics:* Not approved for pediatric use
	Gadodiamide (Omniscan [GE Healthcare]) 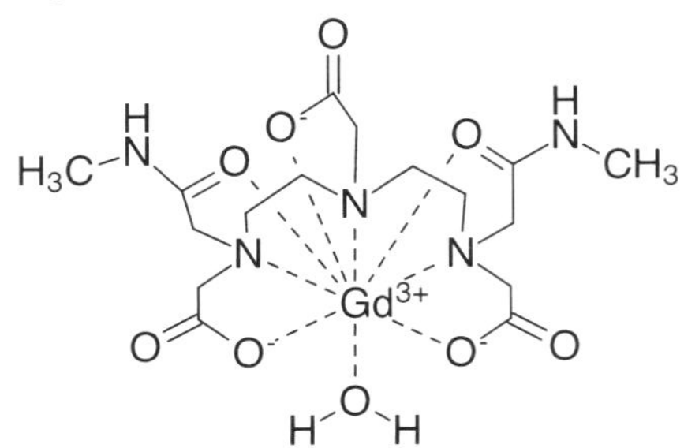	*CNS:* 0.2 mL/kg (0.1 mmol/kg) as bolus IV injection; may be followed with second dose of 0.4 mL/kg (0.2 mmol/kg) within 20 minutes after first dose *Kidney:* 0.1 mL/kg (0.05 mmol/kg) *Abdominal/Thoracic (Noncardiac)/Pelvic:* 0.2 mL/kg (0.1 mmol/kg) *Pediatrics (2–16 years of age):* *CNS:* 0.2 mL/kg (0.1 mmol/kg) as bolus IV injection *Kidney:* 0.1 mL mL/kg (0.05 mmol/kg)

		Abdominal/Thoracic (Noncardiac)/Pelvic: 0.2 mL/kg (0.1 mmol/kg)
Ionic, linear	Gadopentetate dimeglumine (Magnevist [Bayer Healthcare]) 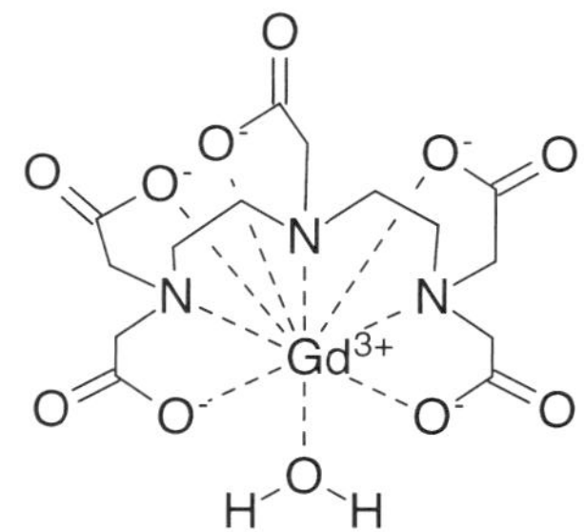	*CNS/Extracranial/Extraspinal Tissues/Body:* 0.2 mL/kg (0.1 mmol/kg) at rate no greater than 10 mL per 15 seconds *Pediatrics (2 years of age and older):* *CNS/Extracranial/Extraspinal Tissues/Body:* 0.2 mL/kg (0.1 mmol/kg) at rate no greater than 10 mL per 15 seconds
Nonionic, cyclic	Gadoteridol (ProHance [Bracco Diagnostics]) 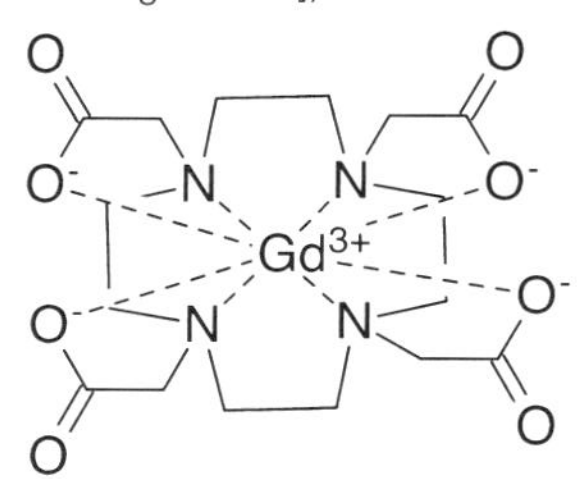	*CNS:* 0.2 mL/kg (0.1 mmol/kg) as rapid IV infusion (10–60 mL/min) or by bolus IV injection (>60 mL/min); may be followed with second dose of 0.4 mL/kg (0.2 mmol/kg) within 30 minutes of first dose *Extracranial/Extraspinal Tissues:* 0.2 mL/kg (0.1 mmol/kg) as rapid IV infusion (10–60 mL/min) or by bolus IV injection (>60 mL/min) *Pediatrics (2–18 years of age):* *CNS:* 0.2 mL/kg (0.1 mmol/kg) as rapid IV infusion (10–60 mL/min) or by bolus IV injection (>60 mL/min)
Ionic, cyclic	Gadoterate dimeglumine	Not available in United States

so it is excreted primarily via the kidneys, with a very small percentage excreted in the feces.[18]

Table 10-2 provides current dosing guidelines for the high-relaxivity preparations that are currently available in the United States.

Adverse Reactions

Gadolinium contrast agents are well tolerated by most patients receiving them. The occurrence of adverse reactions varies from 0.07% to 2.4% in patients injected with 0.1–0.2 mmol/kg of a gadolinium chelate. The vast majority of reactions are considered mild; some examples are cold feeling at the injection site, headache, dizziness, itching, and paresthesias. The occurrence of a severe nonallergic anaphylactic or anaphylactoid reaction is extremely rare.[19]

Risk factors for acute adverse reactions include history of previous reaction to a gadolinium-containing contrast agent, asthma, and allergic reactions to other medicines or foods.[19] Even with pretreatment with corticosteroids and antihistamines, allergylike reactions may still take place.[20] For moderate or severe acute adverse reactions to gadolinium contrast agents, treatment is similar to that provided for moderate to severe acute reactions resulting from administration of iodinated contrast media.[19]

Penfield and Reilly[21] reported that the administration of gadolinium chelates can result in acute kidney damage, particularly with the high doses necessary for angiography. In addition, they stated that artifacts connected with the administration of gadolinium could occur with several laboratory tests, the most significant problem being pseudohypocalcemia. The probability of these latter two adverse reactions becomes greater with declining renal function.[21]

In May 2007, the Food and Drug Administration (FDA) called for manufacturers of all gadolinium-containing contrast agents to add a boxed warning to their labeling for patients with acute or chronic severe renal insufficiency, those with acute renal insufficiency of any severity resulting from hepatorenal syndrome, and those in the perioperative liver transplantation time frame. In these patient populations, there is increased risk of developing nephrogenic systemic fibrosis (NSF) upon exposure to gadolinium-based contrast agents. In postmarketing reports, it has been shown that NSF can occur following single or multiple administrations of gadolinium contrast agents.[22]

Table 10-2. High-Relaxivity Gadolinium Contrast Agents[3,13,14,16]

Agent	Dosing
Gadobenate dimeglumine (MultiHance [Bracco Diagnostics]) 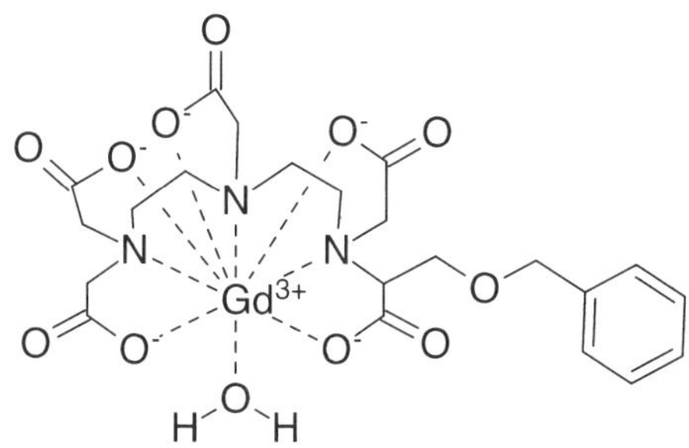	*Central nervous system:* 0.2 mL/kg (0.1 mmol/kg) as rapid bolus IV injection *Pediatrics:* Not approved for pediatric use
Gadofosveset trisodium (Ablavar [Lantheus Medical Imaging]) 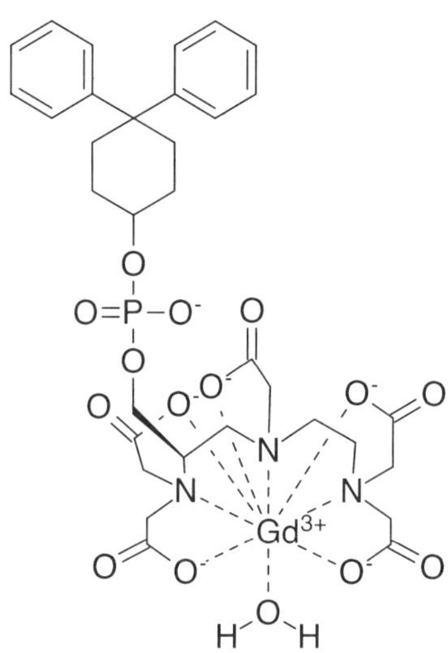	*Magnetic resonance angiography:* 0.12 mL/kg (0.03 mmol/kg) over 30 seconds or less *Pediatrics:* Not approved for pediatric use

(*continued*)

Table 10-2. High-Relaxivity Gadolinium Contrast Agents[3,13,14,16] (*Continued*)

Agent	Dosing
Gadoxetate disodium (Eovist [Bayer Healthcare]) 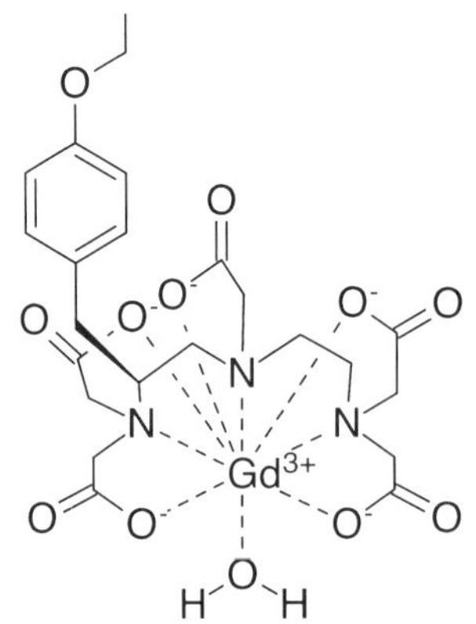	*Liver:* 0.1 mL/kg (0.025 mmol/kg) by bolus IV injection at approximately 2 mL/sec *Pediatrics:* Not approved for pediatric use

In September 2010, FDA required a new warning on the labels of gadolinium-based contrast agents regarding the risk and potentially fatal outcome if these contrast agents are given to certain patients with kidney disease. According to a September 2010 FDA news release, three gadolinium-based contrast media (Magnevist, Omniscan, and Optimark) are contraindicated for use in patients with acute kidney injury or chronic, severe kidney disease.[23] However, labels for all gadolinium-based contrast agents must emphasize the necessity of screening patients to identify these types of kidney dysfunction prior to administration. Table 10-3 lists additional FDA recommendations to health care professionals regarding the use of these imaging agents.

NSF is described as a fibrosing disease, predominantly detected in the subcutaneous tissues and skin, but this disease can be found in other organs, such as the skeletal muscles, heart, eyes, joints, esophagus, and lungs.[19,22,23] NSF usually involves the upper and lower extremities, with the trunk involved less frequently.[6] After signs and symptoms develop, they can quickly advance, with some affected individuals progressing to joint immobility and contractures[19] as a result of skin tightening and hardening. The time between administration of a gadolinium-based

Table 10-3. FDA Safety Recommendations for Use of Gadolinium-Based Contrast Media[23]

Do not use Magnevist, Omniscan, or Optimark in patients having acute kidney injury or chronic, severe kidney disease.
Perform laboratory testing to estimate kidney function in patients at risk for chronically reduced kidney function.
Avoid the use of gadolinium-based contrast agents in patients known or suspected to have impaired drug elimination, unless the imaging procedure is a necessity and is not available without administration of a contrast agent.
Monitor patients who are known or suspected to have impaired renal elimination for signs and symptoms of nephrogenic systemic fibrosis after administration of a gadolinium-based contrast agent.
Administer gadolinium-based contrast media only one time during an imaging session.

contrast agent and diagnosis of NSF has ranged from a few days to several months.[6] A fatal outcome is possible, and this is thought to be due to involvement of visceral organs.[19] The etiology of this disease is not known, but in recent years it has been reported in severe renal insufficiency patients who are administered gadolinium-containing contrast media. It should be noted, however, that cases have been reported in the medical literature in patients without known exposure to these agents.[6]

Contraindications

According to the boxed warning found on all gadolinium products, these agents should be avoided in any patient with acute or chronic severe renal insufficiency or renal insufficiency associated with hepatorenal syndrome and in the perioperative liver transplantation period unless the diagnostic information to be obtained is essential.[22] FDA has stated that the use of Magnevist, Omniscan, and Optimark in patients with acute kidney injury or chronic severe kidney disease is contraindicated; all patients who are to receive gadolinium-based contrast agents are required to be screened for these types of kidney disease.[23] Other contraindications to gadolinium contrast agents include a history of prior allergic or hypersensitivity reactions to gadolinium contrast agents or to any components of the products.[9,12,13]

Medication Therapy Management (MTM) Concerns

Gadobenate dimeglumine is a substrate for the canalicular multispecific organic anion transporter (cMOAT), so it has the possibility of competing with other drugs that utilize this anionic transporter. Examples of drugs that are substrates for cMOAT are cisplatin, anthracyclines, vincristine, methotrexate, etoposide, tamoxifen, and paclitaxel. Also, anionic drugs that are excreted in bile (e.g., rifampicin) may decrease the hepatic contrast effects and biliary excretion of gadoxetate. Administration of gadodiamide and gadoversetamide has been shown to interfere with serum calcium measurements, producing a falsely low serum calcium value if the sample is taken before the agent is completely cleared from the body; the other nonspecific agents do not interfere with this measurement. In patients who have recently received gadodiamide or gadoversetamide, this interaction should be considered before supplemental calcium is administered to correct the apparent deficiency. Gadoxetate may alter serum iron levels for up to 24 hours after administration, and gadopentetate dimeglumine can produce transitory alterations in serum iron, transaminase, and bilirubin levels.[6]

Superparamagnetic Contrast Agents

Superparamagnetic iron oxides (SPIOs or ferumoxides) and ultrasmall superparamagnetic iron oxides (USPIOs) constitute this group of contrast agents. These agents have an iron oxide core (diameter of 3 to 5 nm) enclosed in a low molecular weight dextran or carbodextran, depending on the product. The dextran and carbodextran prevent the magnetic crystals from undergoing uncontrolled aggregation. The theory behind the design of these agents is that smaller particles have a longer circulation time in the blood and may collect in the macrophages of the liver, spleen, and lymph nodes, whereas the larger particles target particularly the hepatic tissue and also have a reduced half-life in the blood.[3]

The indication for SPIOs is liver imaging.[3] The USPIOs are being evaluated for MR lymphography,[3] and they are not available for clinical use in the United States.

Conclusion

Paramagnetic and superparamagnetic contrast agents enhance the diagnostic utility of MR imaging, and new agents are being developed to further the usefulness of this imaging modality. Knowledge of possible drug interactions with these agents and the potential for alteration of laboratory test values will assist pharmacists in providing improved pharmaceutical care. It is critical for patients to be screened for possible contraindications and health risks through review of their medical and drug history.

References

1. Jackels SC. Enhancement agents for magnetic resonance imaging: fundamentals. In: Swanson DP, Chilton HM, Thrall JH, eds. *Pharmaceuticals in Medical Imaging.* New York: Macmillan; 1990:645–61.
2. Jensen SC, Peppers MP. Classification, chemistry, and pharmacology of contrast agents. In: Jensen SC, Peppers MP, eds. *Pharmacology and Drug Administration for Imaging Technologists.* 2nd ed. St Louis: Mosby Elsevier; 2006:64–80.
3. Aspelin P, Bellin MF, Jakobsen JA, et al. Classification and terminology. In: Thomsen HS, Webb JAW, eds. *Medical Radiology Diagnostic Imaging: Contrast Media Safety Issues and ESUR Guidelines.* 2nd ed. Berlin, Heidelberg: Springer-Verlag; 2009:3–9.
4. Saini S, Ferrucci JT. Enhancement agents for magnetic resonance imaging: clinical applications. In: Swanson DP, Chilton HM, Thrall JH, eds. *Pharmaceuticals in Medical Imaging.* New York: Macmillan; 1990:645–61.
5. Caravan P. Strategies for increasing the sensitivity of gadolinium based MRI contrast agents. *Chem Soc Rev.* 2006;35:512–23.
6. American Society of Health-System Pharmacists. Quick Guide to Contrast Media. Developed by ASHP Advantage. www.ashp.org/Import/PRACTICEANDPOLICY/PracticeResourceCenters/ContrastMedia/QuickGuidetoContrastMedia.aspx. Accessed September 15, 2010.
7. Weinmann H-J, Brasch RC, Press W-R, et al. Characteristics of gadolinium-DTPA complex: a potential NMR contrast agent. *AJR Am J Roentgenol.* 1984;142:619–24.
8. OptiMark [package insert]. St. Louis: Mallinckrodt; 2009.
9. Omniscan [package insert]. Princeton, NJ: GE Healthcare; 2007.
10. Magnevist [package insert]. Wayne, NJ: Bayer HealthCare Pharmaceuticals; 2010.
11. ProHance [package insert]. Princeton, NJ: Bracco Diagnostics; 2007.
12. Bellin MF, Vasile M, Morel-Precetti S. Currently used non-specific extracellular MR contrast media. *Eur Radiol.* 2003;13:2688–98.
13. Eovist [package insert]. Wayne, NJ: Bayer HealthCare Pharmaceuticals; 2008.
14. MultiHance Multipack [package insert]. Princeton, NJ: Bracco Diagnostics; 2009.
15. Gadofosveset. Drugdex Evaluations, Micromedex Healthcare series. www.thomsonhc.com. Accessed May 6, 2010 (access available only to subscribers).
16. Ablavar [package insert]. Billerica, MA: Lantheus Medical Imaging; 2009.
17. Gadoxetate. Drugdex Evaluations, Micromedex Healthcare series. www.thomsonhc.com. Accessed May 6, 2010 (access available only to subscribers).
18. Gadobenate Dimeglumine. Drugdex Evaluations, Micromedex Healthcare series. www.thomsonhc.com. Accessed May 6, 2010 (access available only to subscribers).
19. American College of Radiology Committee on Drugs and Contrast Media. Manual on Contrast Media v.7.0. 2010.
20. Heinz-Peer G. Acute adverse reactions. In: Thomsen HS, Webb JAW, eds. *Medical Radiology Diagnostic Imaging: Contrast Media Safety Issues and ESUR Guidelines.* 2nd ed. Berlin, Heidelberg: Springer-Verlag; 2009:181–5.

21. Penfield JG, Reilly RF Jr. What nephrologists need to know about gadolinium CME. *Nat Clin Pract Nephrol.* 2007;3:654–68. www.nature.com/nrneph/journal/v3/n12/full/ncpneph0660.html. Accessed September 7, 2011.
22. Food and Drug Administration. Information for healthcare professionals: gadolinium-based contrast agents for magnetic resonance imaging. June 2006, updated December 2006 and May 23, 2007. www.fda.gov/Drugs/DrugSafety/PostmarketDrugSafetyInformationforPatientsandProviders/ucm142884.htm. Accessed September 23, 2011.
23. Food and Drug Administration. FDA drug safety communication: new warnings for using gadolinium-based contrast agents in patients with kidney dysfunction [news release]. September 9, 2010.

CHAPTER 11

Review of Imaging Procedures Using Ultrasound

Hal J. Minnigan

History and Early Use

Ultrasound is a powerful and safe modality for both diagnostic and therapeutic use in modern medicine. Its origins can be traced to the development of an understanding of the properties of sound waves and the principle of the echo. In the mid 18th century, Spallanzani demonstrated that bats are blind and navigate by means of echoes of inaudible sound.[1] Half a century later, Christian Johann Doppler described what we now know as the "Doppler effect," namely, that the pitch of a sound varies if the source of the sound is moving.[2] The discovery of the piezoelectric properties of crystals in the late 19th century by the Curies[3] permitted the generation of ultrasonic waves. A great advance in the development of ultrasound imaging came in 1912 when a British engineer, L. F. Richardson, proposed the use of echolocation to detect underwater objects. Subsequently, during World War I an American, Paul Langevin, developed the earliest form of sonar to detect submarines under water. Concurrently, Firestone[4] developed an ultrasonographic technique for imaging metal for purposes of flaw detection in fabricated and welded joints. This embodied the crux of modern-day diagnostic ultrasound: the transmission and reception of sound waves coupled with imaging and location of the target.

Perhaps the first use of ultrasound for medical imaging was in 1941, when an Austrian, Karl Dussik,[5] attempted to image the cerebral ventricles with ultrasound. Between 1947 and 1949 Dr. George D. Ludwig, at the Naval Medical Research Institute, Bethesda, Maryland, and later at the Massachusetts Institute of Technology, demonstrated that gallbladder stones could be detected by an ultrasonic echo method using A-mode metal flaw detectors and naval sonar. The work of Professor Ian Donald and his colleagues in Glasgow in the mid 1950s did much to facilitate the development of practical technology and applications. This led to the wider use of ultrasound in medical practice in subsequent decades. The first recognizable use of ultrasound for cardiac imaging resulted from a collaboration between Hertz and Edler, who in 1953 in Sweden used an industrial test instrument to examine the heart.[6] The development of color flow Doppler, spectral Doppler, and power Doppler imaging was greatly assisted by parallel advances in computer development, which allowed the complex mathematical computations needed to process images to be created and displayed in real time.

Physics of Ultrasound

A brief introduction to the physical principles of ultrasound as it is used in medicine is in order, before discussion of the various ultrasound modalities. Ultrasound is defined as sound waves with frequencies above the audible range, that is, greater than 20 kiloHertz (kHz). Most diagnostic ultrasound uses frequencies from 1 megaHertz (MHz) to about 18 MHz. Ultrasound waves are generated and propagated from the transducer face in a linear fashion, by application of an electric pulse to a piezoelectric substance in the transducer. A piezoelectric substance has the unique property of producing mechanical vibrations when stimulated by an electric current, and vice versa. This allows it to be used in an ultrasound transducer to both "talk" and "listen." When an electrical pulse is applied to the piezoelectric crystal, an ultrasound wave is generated. This wave has properties of wavelength, frequency, and period, as do electromagnetic waves; however, ultrasound waves are physical and longitudinal and do not contain electromagnetic radiation (Figure 11-1).[7] Ultrasound waves returning to the transducer (echoes) strike the piezoelectric crystals and generate an electrical signal that

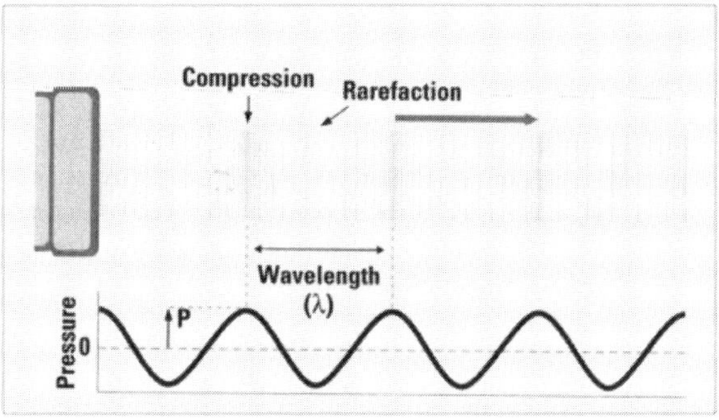

Figure 11-1. Diagrammatic representation of a sound wave with areas of compression and rarefaction. The upper part of the diagram represents the sound wave as a longitudinal wave propagating from the transducer face, diagrammatically showing the areas of compression and rarefaction of the tissue. Below this is a representation of an ultrasound wave as a traditional sine wave, with amplitude and frequency indicated. The areas of compression and rarefaction in the longitudinal wave correspond to the peaks and troughs in the sine wave. (Reprinted with permission from reference 7.)

is converted by the ultrasound machine into the image displayed on the screen.

The basis of diagnostic ultrasound depends on transmission of a brief ultrasound pulse of a few microseconds ("talking"), followed by a period of reception of the returning echoes, which is commonly 100 times longer in duration ("listening"). Generation of a returning echo depends on differences in the interaction of the ultrasound wave with the different types of tissues it comes in contact with. This property, known as acoustic impedance, depends chiefly on the density of the tissue or medium and the speed of the transmitted sound wave. Ultrasound waves have an average speed in soft tissue of 1540 meters per second, but each tissue type conducts ultrasound at different speeds. Most incident ultrasound waves are scattered by the tissue and never return to the transducer, but some are reflected in such a manner as to form an "echo" that is usable in creating an ultrasound signal or image (Figure 11-2).[7] Thus, the ultrasound information is gathered from echoes of different intensities (amplitudes) received at different times after the original pulse is sent. The ultrasound machine processes this information in different ways for display, depending on the mode the user has selected, as described below.

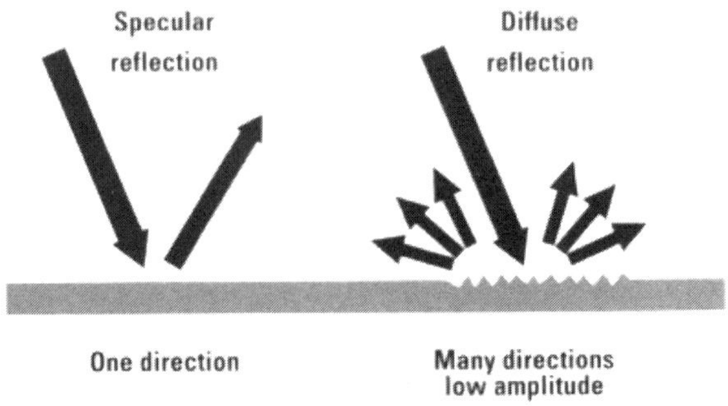

Figure 11-2. Illustration of reflection leading to solitary echo (left), compared with diffuse reflection (right) that leads to loss of most ultrasound energy in the medium. (Reprinted with permission from reference 7.)

The ability of an ultrasound echo to resolve, or discriminate between, very small differences in structure depends on the wavelength of the ultrasound beam and also on a difference in acoustic impedance between the two structures. Higher frequencies have shorter wavelengths; thus, higher-frequency ultrasound waves can resolve smaller differences in tissue. High-frequency ultrasound waves are able to resolve smaller differences in tissue structure but are limited by how far they can penetrate into the tissue. Conversely, lower-frequency ultrasound waves penetrate more deeply into tissue but are unable to provide resolution comparable to that with higher-frequency waves. Thus, resolution and penetration are inversely related.

Ultrasound Modalities

Ultrasound information can be processed in several ways, with results displayed to the user in real time. The different display types are known as "modes." The typical modes are A-mode, B-mode, M-mode, and Doppler ultrasound. Modes vary in terms of the sonic information that the transducer sends out and also in terms of the processing of the information received by the transducer before it is displayed to the operator. Each of these modes is briefly described below.

A-Mode

A-mode was the earliest mode of ultrasound imaging but is rarely used in diagnostic imaging today. A-mode stands for "amplitude mode."

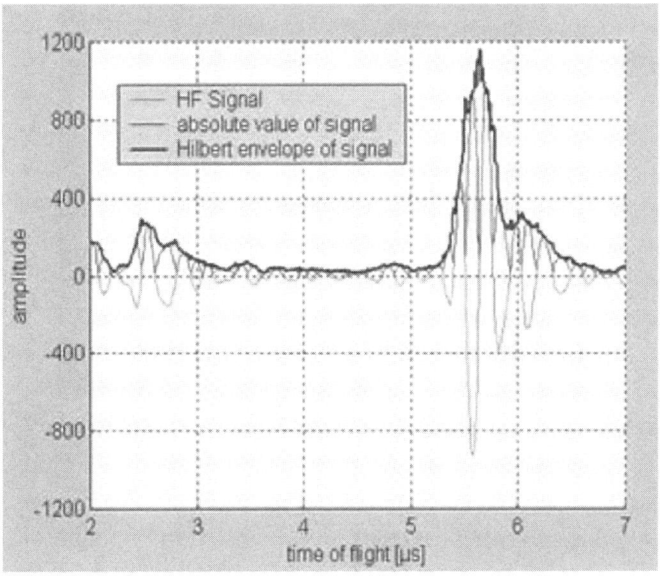

Figure 11-3. (also in color section following page 210) Graphical representation of an A-mode ultrasound. The green tracing is the raw ultrasound signal as it returns echoes to the machine. It is converted to all positive values for display (red tracing). A complex mathematical transformation is performed (the Hilbert transformation), which fits the ultrasound signal to a smoothed curve for display to the user. HF = high-frequency. (Reprinted with permission from reference 7.)

The returning ultrasound echo information is displayed on a graph (Figure 11-3)[7] with the instantaneous amplitude of the returning echoes versus the time after transmission of the acoustical pulse. In this tracing, the time of an echo's return is proportional to its distance in the tissue, so the tracing is also a display of signal amplitude versus depth in the tissue.

B-Mode

B-mode stands for "brightness mode" or 2-D mode, because the image is displayed on a gray-scale image screen in two dimensions, and differentiation of tissues is displayed as varying shades of gray. This is the traditional mode of imaging that most medical professionals think of when they think of ultrasound. The depth of the echo information is plotted in a vertical fashion on the screen, and the intensity of the returning echoes is displayed as shades of gray. The top of the screen usually

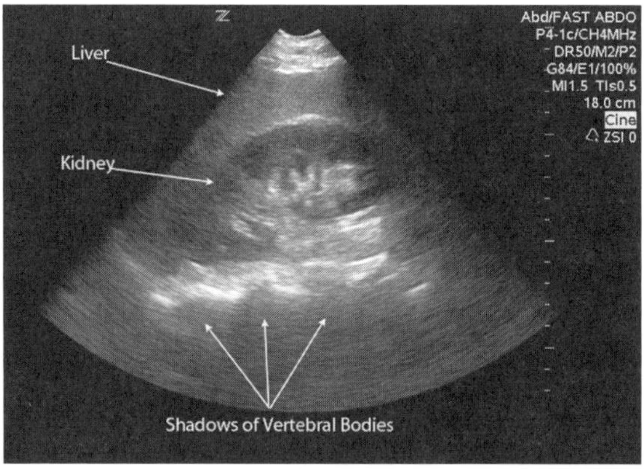

Figure 11-4. Coronal B-mode image of right flank. Labeled structures include the liver, right kidney, and shadow artifacts created by thoracic vertebral bodies.

represents the origin of the sound beam (the transducer face). The depth of the returning echo is represented as an image displayed farther away (farther down on the screen) from the transducer face. Stronger echoes generally are displayed as brighter or whiter on the screen. The screen is refreshed so rapidly (about 30 times per second) that the image is essentially a real-time representation of the tissue being imaged (Figure 11-4). This gives a representation of the anatomic structures being imaged that is a slice through the tissues in the plane of the ultrasound beam. The tools most often used in B-mode imaging are simple tools for measuring distance and volume. B-mode is the standard imaging mode in diagnostic ultrasound today. Other modes of imaging are often used in conjunction with B-mode to gain additional information. For example, in imaging an artery to assess for stenosis or impaired flow, the sonographer uses B-mode imaging to anatomically identify the artery under examination and then uses another mode (e.g., color flow or spectral Doppler) to assess flow abnormalities. Such use of two imaging modes simultaneously is called *duplex imaging*.

M-Mode

M-mode, or "motion mode," is a horizontal linear display of the B-mode information from a single ultrasound beam, which is continuously displayed from left to right across the screen. The structure of interest is located using a B-mode image, and the axis of the M-mode beam

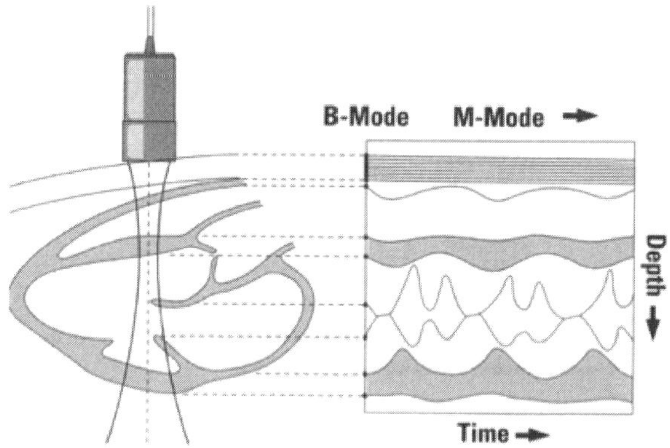

Figure 11-5. Diagrammatic representation of M-mode imaging. The ultrasound beam is held stationary, while the image displays the B-mode information in a real-time left-to-right display of depth versus time as indicated. (Reprinted with permission from reference 7.)

is selected by the sonographer using a cursor on the screen. Moving structures are seen as waves on the horizontal trace that undulate vertically as they move with respect to the ultrasound transducer (Figures 11-5[7] and 11-6). The main use of this modality is in cardiology, to assess cardiac motion.

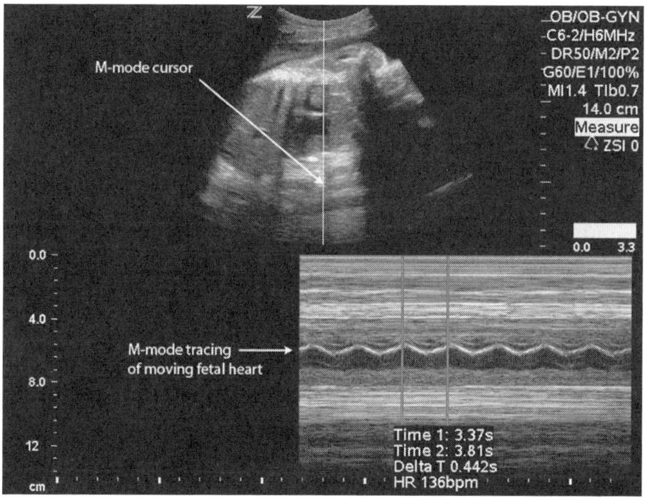

Figure 11-6. (also in color section following page 210) M-mode image of a fetal heart in utero. The labeled M-mode cursor in the upper pane is over the moving heart in the B-mode image. The lower panel shows the M-mode tracing of the moving wall of the fetal heart, with calipers used to calculate the fetal heart rate.

Doppler Ultrasound

Doppler ultrasound comprises three basic modes: color flow, power Doppler, and spectral Doppler. All these modes depend on the Doppler principle, first described by J. C. Doppler in 1842.[8] This principle states that the frequency (pitch) of a sound wave is higher if the source of the sound wave is moving toward the observer and lower if the source of the sound wave is moving away from the observer. In medical ultrasound, the moving structures that are interrogated are red blood cells in vascular structures. The ultrasound machine sends out a pulse of sound waves and listens for the returning echoes. If the returning echoes are at a higher pitch (frequency) than the original ultrasound wave, then the flow of blood is considered to be toward the transducer. If the returning echoes are at a lower pitch (frequency) than the original sound wave, the flow of blood is considered to be away from the transducer. Thus, the frequency shift (or Doppler shift) of the returning echoes provides information about the direction and velocity of the moving red blood cells relative to the transducer.

Color Flow Doppler Mode

In color flow mode, the ultrasound machine can display information about the direction and speed of blood flow. The color red is arbitrarily assigned to flow toward the transducer, and blue is assigned to flow away from the transducer. Differing velocities of flow are displayed on a graduated palette of colors, which is known as a color map (Figure 11-7). The color information is displayed superimposed on the B-mode image, in a so-called duplex imaging mode.

Color Power Doppler Mode

Color power Doppler, a relatively recently developed mode, displays flow with respect to energy, or intensity, but does not display directional information. Color is displayed as varying intensities of one color, often a red-orange color (Figure 11-8). The theoretical advantage of power Doppler mode is that it is more sensitive in detecting low flow, inasmuch as it displays the sum of the energies of the moving reflectors (red blood cells), rather than their velocities. This is helpful when flow is low; thus, power Doppler is often used to find vessels with limited flow, after which other modes can be used to assess the velocity and direction of flow if necessary.

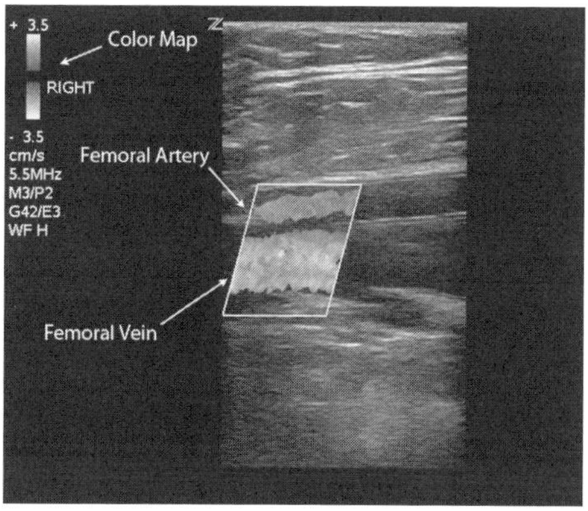

Figure 11-7. (also in color section following page 210) Color flow Doppler image of femoral artery and vein. The red color fills the artery and indicates flow toward the transducer. The vein is colored blue. The color map is indicated in the upper left of the image.

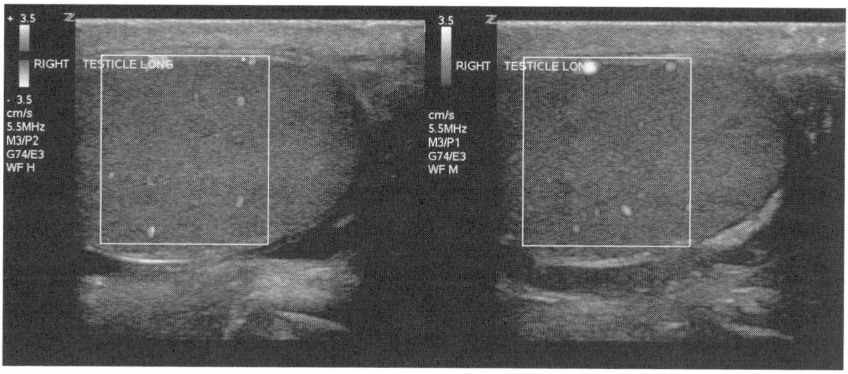

Figure 11-8. (also in color section following page 210) Comparison of color flow Doppler and color power Doppler images. On the left is a color flow image of a testicle. Red and blue color flow are both visible within the testicular parenchyma. On the right is a color power Doppler image of the same testicle. Similar signals are present, but as indicated by the color map on the right panel, all flow is indicated by variations of red/orange color.

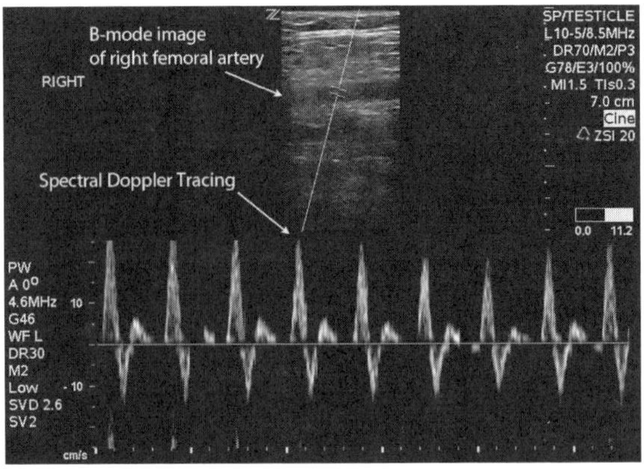

Figure 11-9. Spectral Doppler image of the common femoral artery. The B-mode and spectral Doppler trace are indicated.

Spectral Doppler Mode

Spectral Doppler displays velocity and direction information on a linear trace and provides audible information about the Doppler shift. The instantaneous velocity of flow is displayed on the vertical axis of a trace versus time, below the B-mode image. Flow toward the transducer is displayed above the reference line, and flow away from the transducer is displayed below the reference line (Figure 11-9). The shape of the waveform can be analyzed both visually by the user and mathematically by the machine, permitting calculation of peak velocity of flow as well as flow volume. For example, information about velocity and flow in the carotid artery can be used to clinically assess for stenosis in the carotid.

Equipment Used

Ultrasound machines exist in a wide array of shapes and sizes, some having a very narrow range of intended use and others performing a broad range of functions. Early diagnostic ultrasound machines were large and not portable. Advances in computer technology have allowed size reductions at all levels. All current diagnostic ultrasound machines are portable, ranging from full-size cart-based machines to hand-held portable units. Most ultrasound machines have interchangeable transducers, which are designed for a variety of specific functions. Transducers are designed to transmit and receive the ultrasound pulses

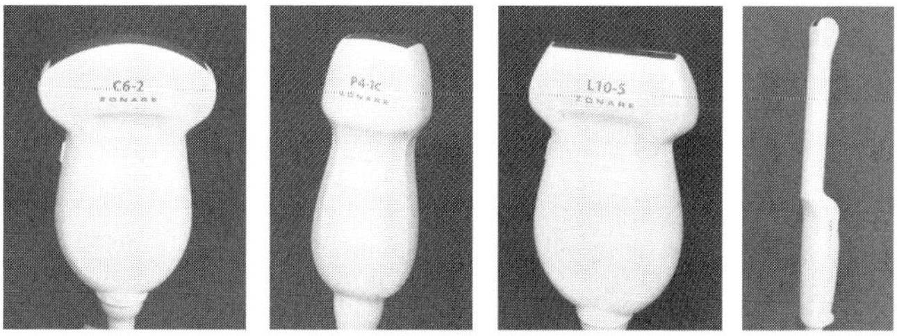

Figure 11-10. Main transducer types used in diagnostic ultrasound (left to right): Curved array transducer used for general abdominal imaging, phased array transducer primarily used for cardiac imaging, high-frequency linear array transducer used for vascular and small-parts imaging, and endocavitary transducer used for endovaginal and endorectal imaging.

and interconvert the mechanical and electrical energy via piezoelectric crystals placed just under the transducer face. Representative ultrasound transducers are shown in Figure 11-10.

Safety Issues

In general, ultrasound is considered the safest imaging modality, primarily because it, like magnetic resonance imaging (MRI), does not involve ionizing radiation. Safety issues in diagnostic ultrasound are primarily related to potential tissue injury by thermal and mechanical energy transfer. Particle motion in the tissue can theoretically lead to heating in the tissue. In addition, mechanical forces generated in the tissue by ultrasound have the potential to disrupt tissue through cavitation, the generation of tiny bubbles in the tissue due to dissolved gases. The energy transferred to the tissue in diagnostic ultrasound has never been shown to cause any damage to tissue in vivo. The guiding principle for acoustic exposure in diagnostic ultrasound is "ALARA," an acronym for "as low as reasonably achievable."[9] This principle states that the operator should attempt to limit the patient's acoustic exposure by all means possible, that is, by limiting the examination time and by using modes and settings that minimize the exposure. For example, B-mode is generally considered one of the lowest exposure modes, although mathematically M-mode provides the lowest exposure. Color flow Doppler and power Doppler involve significantly higher levels of energy.

Applications of Ultrasound

Cardiology

Arguably, the first uses of diagnostic ultrasound were in imaging the heart.[10] The development of imaging modes for moving structures has given physicians the ability to look at the heart reliably in real time. Echocardiography is the mainstay of diagnostic and noninvasive cardiology. Transthoracic echo is used for evaluation of virtually all aspects of cardiac function except coronary artery function, which can be imaged by tiny transducers placed inside the coronary arteries. Transthoracic echo is used to assess global heart function in both systole and diastole. It can image specific areas of the myocardium that are not contracting in coordination with the rest of the heart. Such focal wall motion abnormalities are suggestive of current or previous infarction or, if shown through a stress test to be reversible, are suggestive of areas of the myocardium perfused by stenotic vessels. Transthoracic echo also provides useful information about function of the valves. Using a combination of the modes previously described (M-mode and Doppler), one can evaluate valves for regurgitation (leakage) and for stenosis (restriction of flow). Echo is often performed for evaluation of the heart for shunts—inappropriate flow from one side of the heart to the other, causing undesirable mixing of oxygenated and unoxygenated blood. This can be done using commercial ultrasound contrast media (see Chapter 12), but often it is done by agitating air into tiny bubbles that are injected into a vein. A mixture of saline and entrained microbubbles is pumped through the heart and is visible on echo as a diffuse reflection or scattering, that is, a white cloudy signal. Assessment of the pericardial space is performed to evaluate for fluid, which can impair the filling of the right side of the heart if it builds up rapidly or to a large volume (see emergency medicine applications, below). Masses in the heart are uncommon but, when present, are often serious; heart masses are usually identifiable with echo. Similarly, clot formation or migration to the heart has potentially serious consequences if the clot embolizes in the right-sided circulation (pulmonary embolism) or the left-sided circulation (stroke or peripheral arterial occlusion). Transesophageal echo (TEE) involves a small steerable transducer, shaped like an endoscope, inserted through the mouth and into the esophagus.

Emergency Medicine, Surgery, Critical Care, and Anesthesia

The uses of ultrasound in these specialties overlap but fall generally into two categories: (1) use of focused ultrasound in the real-time evaluation of a critically ill or decompensated patient and (2) use of ultrasound for procedural guidance in real time. The use of ultrasound in emergency medicine and surgery originated in Europe and Asia, where ultrasound was used in the evaluation of trauma patients.[11] The initial use of ultrasound to evaluate the abdomen and pericardial space for traumatic bleeding gained popularity in the 1980s and was shown to have benefit both in patients with penetrating trauma and in those with blunt trauma.[12–14] The FAST exam (focused assessment with sonography for trauma) has become a standard part of the trauma exam in emergency departments. Ultrasound is used in emergency departments for evaluation of bleeding in the chest (hemothorax) as well as for traumatic bleeding in the abdomen. In addition, an acutely ill trauma patient can be evaluated for pneumothorax with bedside ultrasound. The bedside FAST exam in the emergency department has been modified for use in evaluating patients with undifferentiated shock. Essentially, a focused exam of the heart, lungs, and abdomen is performed to search for acute, reversible or treatable causes of shock. These include cardiac causes (acute myocardial infarction, pericardial tamponade, severe decompensated heart failure, pulmonary embolism, severe volume depletion), pulmonary causes (tension pneumothorax), and abdominal catastrophe (ruptured spleen, leaking abdominal aortic aneurysm, ruptured ectopic pregnancy [Figure 11-11]).

The concept of bedside ultrasound for critically ill patients has found favor in medical and surgical intensive care units; primarily, cardiac and pulmonary exams are used in noninvasive evaluation of patients. This same strategy can be used in the operating room by anesthesiologists to help manage patients under general anesthesia.

Bedside ultrasound is also commonly used to provide guidance during procedures performed in the management of critically ill patients. Traditionally, the use of ultrasound to locate and assist in drainage of fluid collections has been done by radiology departments. Similarly, interventional radiologists have used ultrasound for guidance in placing venous and arterial catheters in anatomically challenging patients (Figure 11-12). Increasingly, emergency physicians, surgeons, intensivists, and anesthesiologists are using ultrasound to safely guide bedside

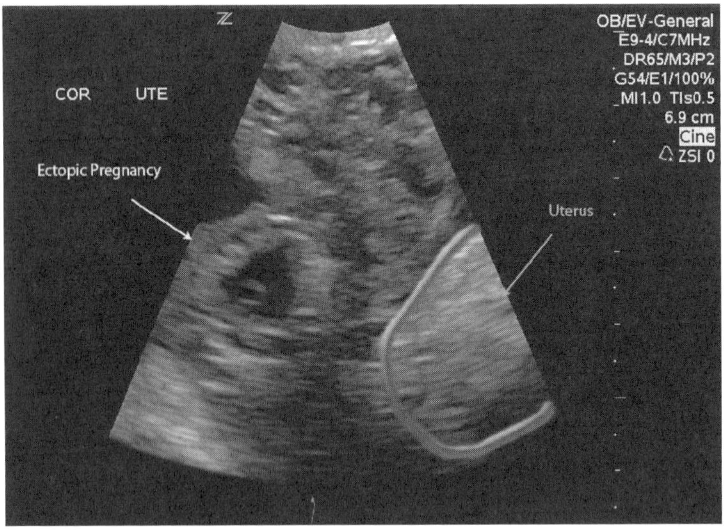

Figure 11-11. (also in color section following page 210) Endovaginal ultrasound image of ruptured right adnexal ectopic pregnancy. The ectopic pregnancy appears as an echogenic (white) ring structure, clearly separated from the uterus.

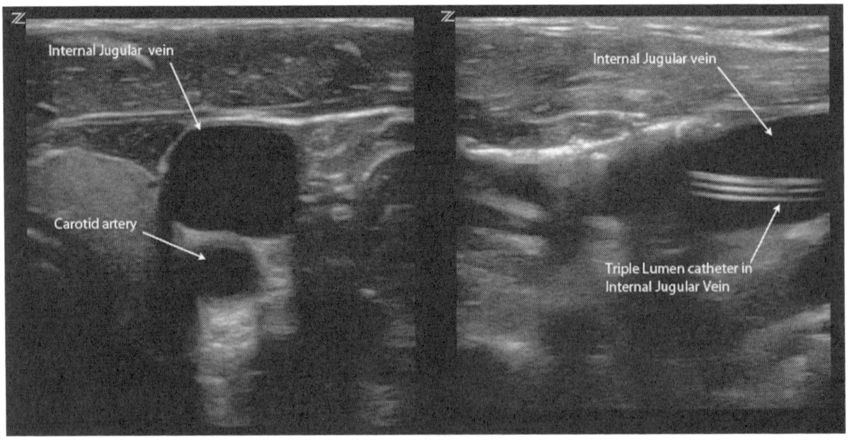

Figure 11-12. B-mode ultrasound images of internal jugular vein. Left panel shows a short-axis (transverse) image of the right internal jugular vein before cannulation for intravenous access. The right panel shows a long-axis image of the same vein after insertion of a triple-lumen central venous catheter under ultrasound guidance.

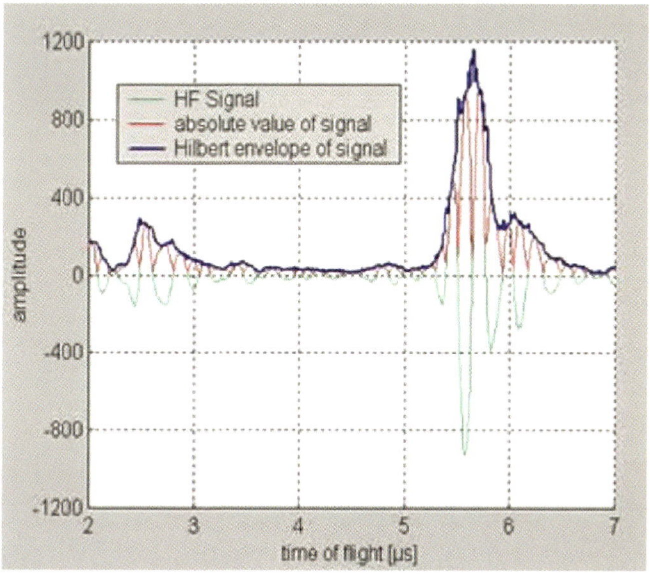

Figure 11-3. Graphical representation of an A-mode ultrasound. The green tracing is the raw ultrasound signal as it returns echoes to the machine. It is converted to all positive values for display (red tracing). A complex mathematical transformation is performed (the Hilbert transformation), which fits the ultrasound signal to a smoothed curve for display to the user. HF = high-frequency. (Reprinted with permission from reference 7.)

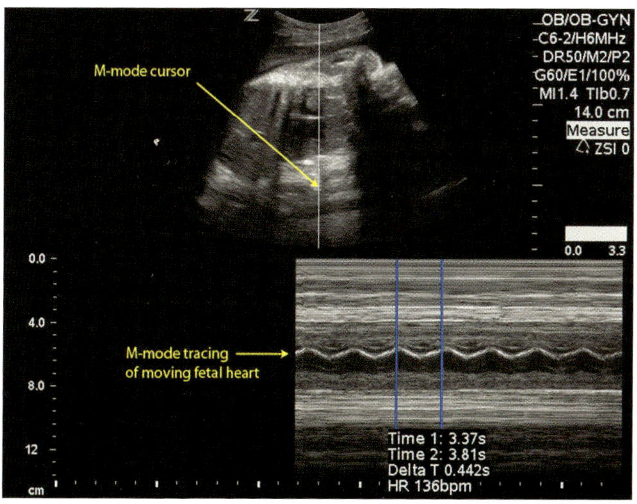

Figure 11-6. M-mode image of a fetal heart in utero. The labeled M-mode cursor in the upper pane is over the moving heart in the B-mode image. The lower panel shows the M-mode tracing of the moving wall of the fetal heart, with calipers used to calculate the fetal heart rate.

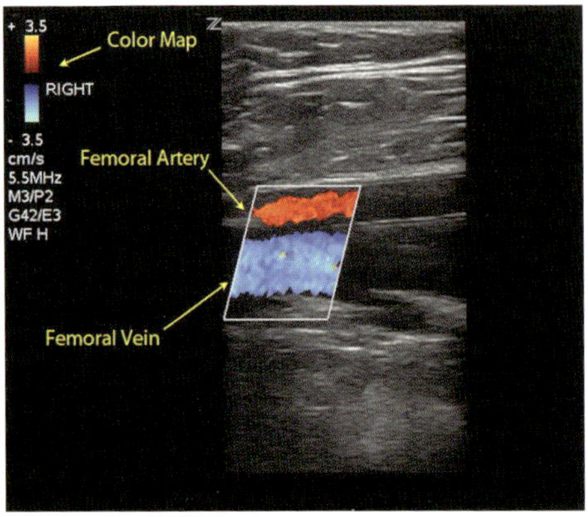

Figure 11-7. Color flow Doppler image of femoral artery and vein. The red color fills the artery and indicates flow toward the transducer. The vein is colored blue. The color map is indicated in the upper left of the image.

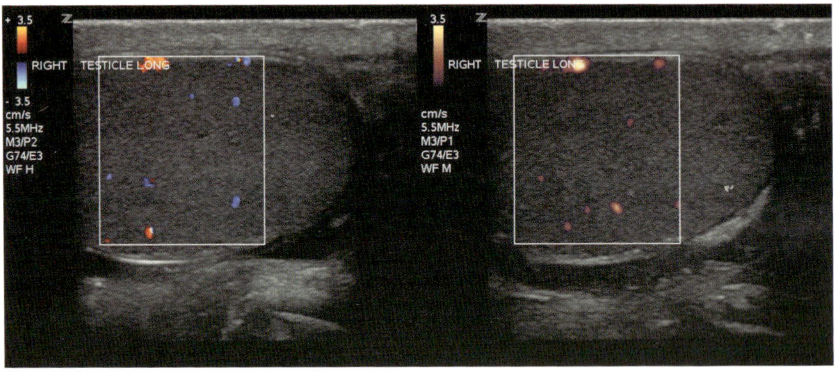

Figure 11-8. Comparison of color flow Doppler and color power Doppler images. On the left is a color flow image of a testicle. Red and blue color flow are both visible within the testicular parenchyma. On the right is a color power Doppler image of the same testicle. Similar signals are present, but as indicated by the color map on the right panel, all flow is indicated by variations of red/orange color.

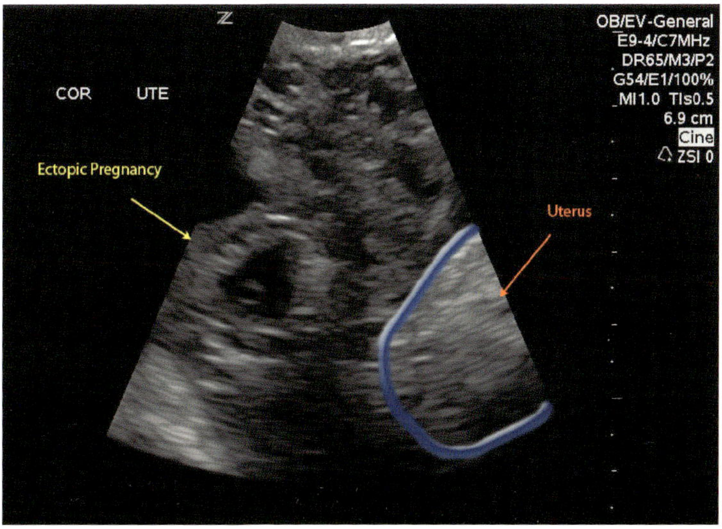

Figure 11-11. Endovaginal ultrasound image of ruptured right adnexal ectopic pregnancy. The ectopic pregnancy appears as an echogenic (white) ring structure, clearly separated from the uterus.

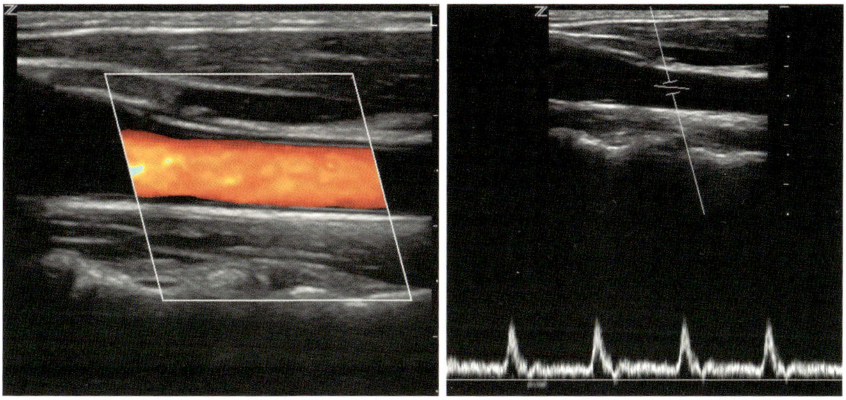

Figure 11-15. Ultrasound images of normal carotid artery. Left panel shows color flow Doppler image of carotid artery. The arterial blood flow in the artery is represented by the orange color. Right panel shows spectral Doppler waveform of the same carotid artery, with a normal arterial waveform at the bottom of the panel.

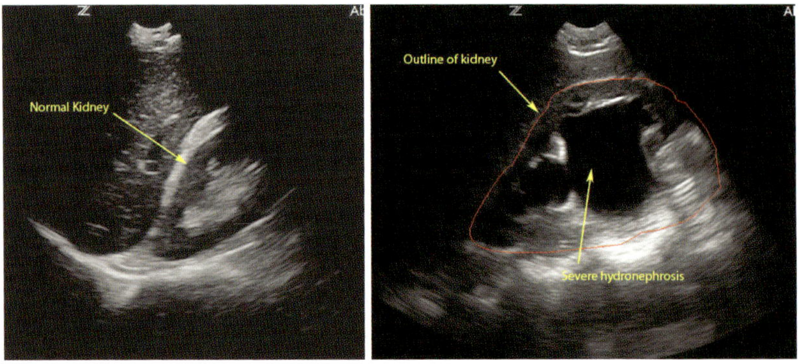

Figure 11-16. Left panel shows ultrasound image of normal kidney. Right panel shows ultrasound image of severe hydronephrosis due to bladder outlet obstruction secondary to prostatic hypertrophy. The anechoic area in the central part of the kidney represents a severely dilated renal collecting system.

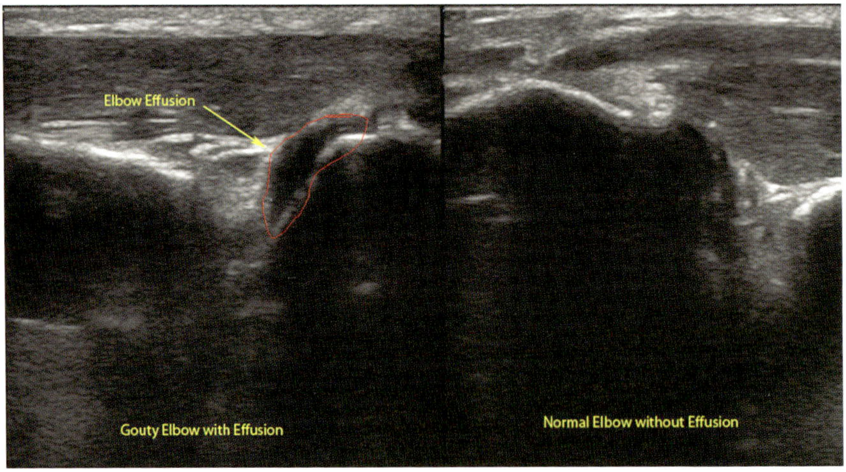

Figure 11-17. Left panel shows ultrasound image of elbow joint with effusion (indicated by arrow). Right panel shows normal elbow without effusion.

procedures. This use of ultrasound for procedural guidance extends to diagnostic and therapeutic drainage of fluid collection from the heart (pericardiocentesis), chest cavity (thoracentesis), and abdomen (paracentesis), as well as joint aspiration (arthrocentesis).

Gastrointestinal

Traditionally, transabdominal ultrasound has been used to evaluate the liver and biliary tract, including gallbladder evaluation for gallstones (Figure 11-13), masses, and infection. Recently, endoscopic ultrasound has come into play as a relatively noninvasive method of imaging and evaluating the gastrointestinal and biliary tracts for masses and stones. Both modalities can be used to evaluate and follow chronic liver disease. The use of ultrasound contrast media has augmented the ability of ultrasound to evaluate flow abnormalities in the portal system that are a consequence of cirrhosis.

Obstetrics and Gynecology

Ultrasound, via both the transabdominal and the endovaginal approach, is a mainstay in the noninvasive evaluation and monitoring of pregnancy (Figure 11-14). Advances in the use of bedside ultrasound in emergency medicine and acute care to confirm the location of an early pregnancy are aimed at reducing the morbidity associated with extrauterine (ectopic) pregnancy.

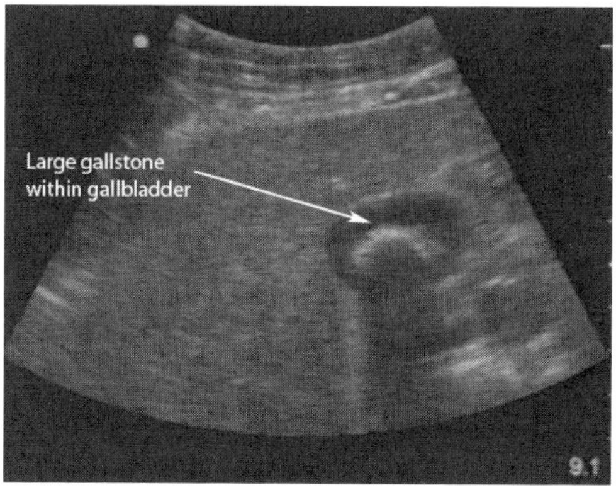

Figure 11-13. Ultrasound image of gallbladder with solitary gallstone and shadowing underneath.

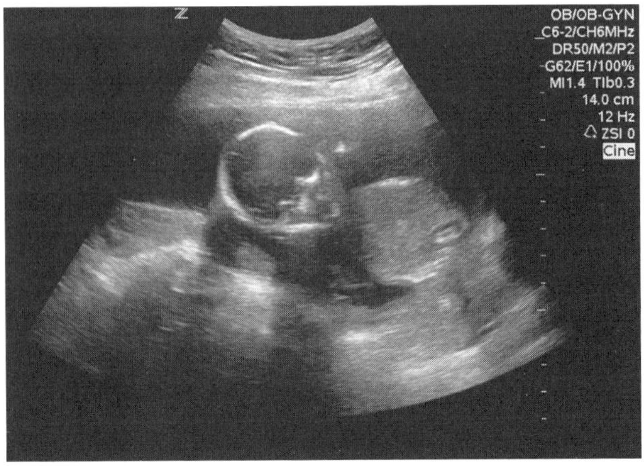

Figure 11-14. Ultrasound image of an approximately 16-week gestational age pregnancy. The head and face are easily recognizable on the left.

Ultrasound was used early in the field of obstetrics, and today advances in ultrasound imaging are used to great advantage to monitor the progress of fetal development in high-risk cases and follow congenital abnormalities. Although there is controversy about the utility of routine screening, most physicians rely on the ability of ultrasound to detect developmental abnormalities so that proper planning and guidance can take place.[15] New technology and understanding have greatly expanded the use of fetal echocardiography, which is immensely helpful in the complex planning process that must take place when a fetal cardiac anomaly is present. Gynecologic uses of ultrasound include evaluation of the ovaries and fallopian tubes, menstrual bleeding problems, and benign and malignant uterine masses.

Neurology

The most common use of ultrasound in neurology is in the evaluation of patients at risk for or suspected of having a stroke. Evaluation of the flow in the carotid arteries can suggest stenosis or dissection (Figure 11-15). The heart also is commonly imaged with ultrasound to look for valvular vegetations as a source of potential emboli and for intracardiac clots and shunts. Although there have been numerous attempts to use ultrasound in the simultaneous diagnostic and therapeutic treatment of thrombotic stroke, favorable outcomes in trials to date have been limited.[16]

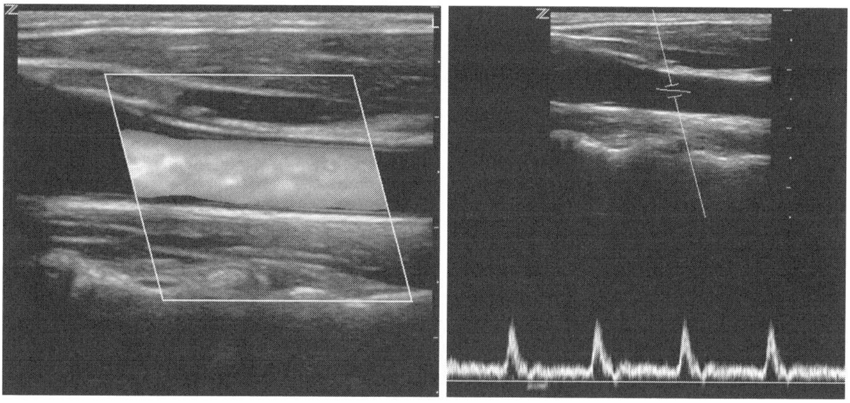

Figure 11-15. (also in color section following page 210) Ultrasound images of normal carotid artery. Left panel shows color flow Doppler image of carotid artery. The arterial blood flow in the artery is represented by the orange color. Right panel shows spectral Doppler waveform of the same carotid artery, with a normal arterial waveform at the bottom of the panel.

Urology

The first use of ultrasound for urologic imaging was in 1961, when Schlegel[17] reported the use of ultrasound to detect renal calculi. Diagnostic ultrasound has a plethora of uses in urologic practice. The kidneys, bladder, prostate, and testicles are all routinely imaged for masses (Figure 11-16). Vascular flow studies are commonly performed

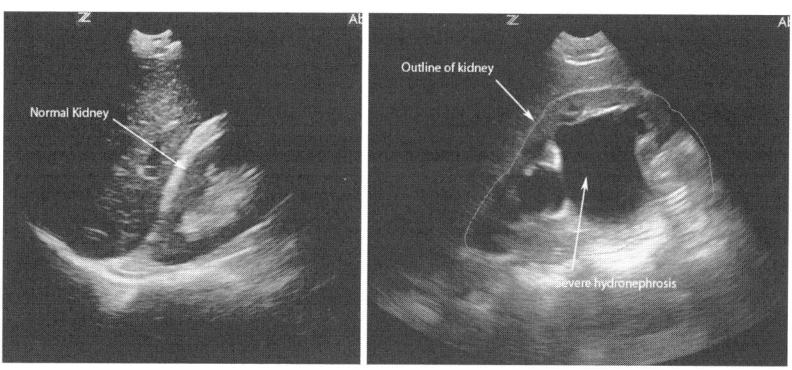

Figure 11-16. (also in color section following page 210) Left panel shows ultrasound image of normal kidney. Right panel shows ultrasound image of severe hydronephrosis due to bladder outlet obstruction secondary to prostatic hypertrophy. The anechoic area in the central part of the kidney represents a severely dilated renal collecting system.

to evaluate the kidneys and testicles. Endoscopic ultrasound can be used to evaluate the urethra and bladder for abnormalities. Renal transplant services often use ultrasound to evaluate a transplanted kidney, which is well positioned for ultrasound imaging, being located in the iliac fossa. Therapeutic urologic ultrasound is discussed below (see Lithotripsy).

Musculoskeletal

Musculoskeletal ultrasound is one of the fastest growing applications of ultrasound, often being performed in the clinic setting as well as in the more traditional radiology suite setting. Ultrasound is used for musculoskeletal imaging in orthopedics, sports medicine, physiatry, and osteopathy. Ultrasound has great utility in imaging muscles and their tendinous insertions, and in some cases it is preferable to MRI. Unlike MRI, ultrasound examination can be performed during movement of a joint, enabling information to be gained for real-time evaluation. Joint effusions (Figure 11-17) are imaged easily with ultrasound, and diagnostic joint aspirations as well as joint injections can be guided by ultrasound. Soft-tissue fluid collections can be localized and drained using ultrasound in real time.

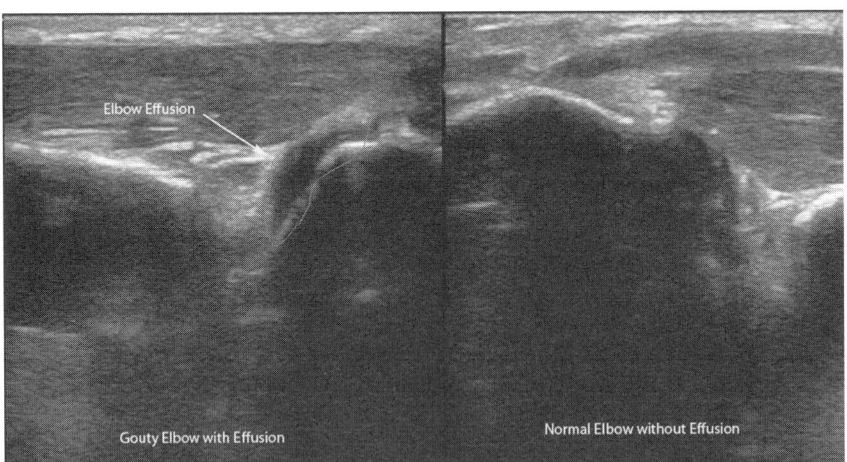

Figure 11-17. (also in color section following page 210) Left panel shows ultrasound image of elbow joint with effusion (indicated by arrow). Right panel shows normal elbow without effusion.

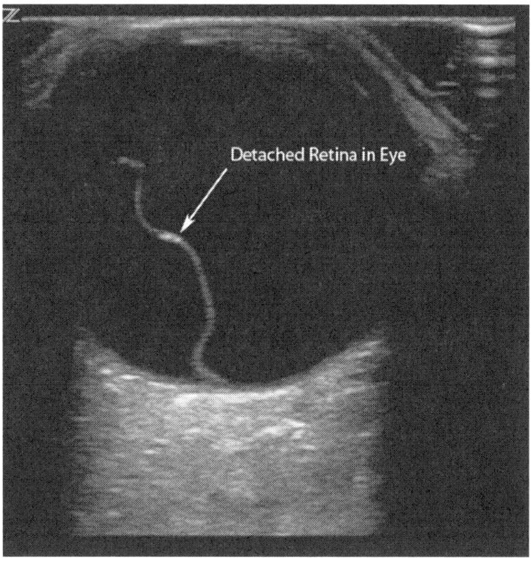

Figure 11-18. Ultrasound image of retinal detachment. A portion of the detached retina is indicated by the arrow.

Ocular

Ultrasound can be used to advantage in evaluation of patients with both nontraumatic and traumatic acute vision loss or change. For example, ultrasound is often used to evaluate an acutely injured eye that may be swollen shut and painful or difficult to open. One of the most common uses of bedside ultrasound in patients with acute eye trauma is in the evaluation of retinal detachment, a time-sensitive and potentially vision-threatening condition (Figure 11-18). In emergency departments and ophthalmology clinics, ocular ultrasound is commonly used to evaluate patients who have vision changes for nontraumatic conditions, including vitreous hemorrhage, vitreous detachment, and spontaneous retinal detachment.

Therapeutic Ultrasound

Lithotripsy

Lithotripsy (extracorporeal shock-wave lithotripsy or ECSWL) uses ultrasound waves to provide acoustic pulses to disrupt a target inside the body, usually renal or gallbladder stones. The patient is positioned on a special bed, which places the acoustic pulse generator near the target tissue. Pulses are generated that enter the body and cause mechanical disruption of the targets by cavitation and shock waves. Heating and patient discomfort are often the limiting factors in this treatment.

Focused Ultrasound Surgery

Focused ultrasound surgery is an evolving technology. It is licensed in the United States for treatment (ablation) of uterine fibroids and in Europe for treatment of painful metastatic bone lesions. It is under investigation for many other applications, including brain tumors, Parkinson's disease, breast cancer, and prostate cancer. The technique currently uses a series of high-intensity ultrasound beams that are independently focused on the lesion of interest. The ultrasound beams are directed at the lesion of interest, often with the use of MRI. The confluence of the ultrasound beams causes highly focused local heating sufficient to cause ablation of the target tissue.

Phacoemulsification

Phacoemulsification is a microscopic ophthalmologic surgical procedure used to remove the lens of the eye, primarily in cataract surgery. During the procedure, a miniature ultrasonic probe is placed inside the capsule holding the lens of the eye. This transducer is then used to emulsify the lens, which is removed by suction or pump during the procedure. A prosthetic lens is then placed inside the lens capsule, which has been preserved. The minimally invasive nature of this procedure allowed by the use of ultrasound contributes to a decrease in pain and postoperative recovery time.

Conclusion

Ultrasound is a portable, noninvasive, and safe imaging modality that is readily available and clinically versatile. Advances in construction and engineering have resulted in smaller and more powerful machines that have found increasing utility outside the radiology and obstetrical suites. New applications in the emergency department and surgical and medical intensive care units extend the utility of ultrasound beyond the traditional radiology and cardiology applications, to include real-time diagnostic and procedural guidance. Outpatient clinics have found ultrasound to be an ideal modality for soft-tissue imaging in musculoskeletal disease. As more clinicians gain expertise in ultrasound, the application of bedside and real-time ultrasound can be expected to facilitate the management of a wide variety of diseases.

References

1. Talbot JH. *A Biographical History of Medicine.* New York: Grune & Stratton; 1935.
2. Feldman A, Ford P. *Scientists and Inventors.* New York: Facts on File; 1979.
3. Curie P, Curie J. Developpement, par pression de l'electricite polaire dans les cristaux hemiedres a faces inclines. *Comptes Rendus.* 1880;91:291.
4. Firestone F, inventor. Flaw-detecting device and measuring instrument. US patent 2,280,226. 1942.
5. Dussik KT. Uber die Moglichkeit Hochfrequente Mechanische schwingungen als Diagnostiches Hilsmittel zu Verwerten. *Z Neurol.* 1941;174:153.
6. Edler I, Hertz CH. Use of ultrasonic reflectoscope for the continuous recording of movements of heart walls. *Kungl Fysiogr Sallsk Lung Forth.* 1954;24:40.
7. Zagzebski J. *Essentials of Ultrasound Physics.* St Louis: Mosby; 1996.
8. Eden A. *The Search for Christian Doppler* [Contains a facsimile edition with an English translation]. Vienna, New York: Springer-Verlag; 1992.
9. *Medical Ultrasound Safety.* Laurel, MD: American Institute of Ultrasound in Medicine; 2009.
10. Armstrong WF, Ryan T. *Feigenbaum's Echocardiography.* Philadelphia: Lippincott, Williams & Wilkins; 2010.
11. Bennett MK, Jehle D. Ultrasonography in blunt abdominal trauma. *Emerg Med Clin North Am.* 1997;15:763–87.
12. Plummer D, Brunette D, Asinger R, et al. Emergency department echocardiography improves outcome in penetrating cardiac injury. *Ann Emerg Med.* 1992;21:709–12.
13. Rozycki GS, Ochsner MG, Jaffin JH, et al. Prospective evaluation of surgeons' use of ultrasound in the evaluation of trauma patients. *J Trauma.* 1993;34:516–26; discussion 526–7.
14. Melniker LA, Leibner E, McKenney MG, et al. Randomized controlled clinical trial of point-of-care, limited ultrasonography for trauma in the emergency department: the first sonography outcomes assessment program trial. *Ann Emerg Med.* 2006;48:227–35.
15. Davey BT, Seubert DE, Phoon CK. Indications for fetal echocardiography high referral, low yield? *Obstet Gynecol Surv.* 2009;64:405–15.
16. Molina CA, Mibo R, Rubiera M, et al. Microbubble administration accelerates clot lysis during continuous 2-MHz ultrasound monitoring in stroke patients treated with intravenous tissue plasminogen activator. *Stroke.* 2006;37:425–9.
17. Schlegel JU, Diggdon P, Cuellar J. The use of ultrasound for localizing renal calculi. *J Urol.* 1961;86:367–9.

CHAPTER 12

Adjunct Agents Used in Ultrasound Imaging

Contrast Media

Jessica Turner

History

Ultrasound contrast media contain small, gas-filled microbubbles that have particular echogenic properties that allow them to be effective enhancers of ultrasound imaging.[1] In the late 1960s, Dr. Charles Joiner was the first to discover that microbubbles could be used for echo-enhancing purposes. While performing an M-mode echocardiogram, Dr. Joiner noticed temporary increases in the ultrasound signal after indocyanine green injections were administered to the patient through a left-ventricular catheter. Further research revealed that the increase in the ultrasound signal was from small air bubbles developing at the catheter tip.[2] Microbubbles were first used as contrast media in echocardiography by Gramiak and Shah in 1968. Normal saline (0.9% sodium chloride) solution was used for intracardiac injections and was shown to improve the definition of the aorta.[1] Although these discoveries were promising, the development of stable microbubbles was essential to ensure their usefulness as contrast agents in ultrasound imaging.

After the discovery that small air bubbles were able to enhance ultrasound imaging, research was conducted to improve the stability and thus the efficacy of the microbubbles. First-generation microbubbles were filled with air and were not stable in circulation after injection because of their high solubility in blood and their consequent short half-life. Also, some of the microbubbles had large diameters, greater than 7 µm, which prevented them from passing through the pulmonary capillary bed. This decreased their effectiveness as contrast agents. To increase their stability, the microbubbles were encased in an outer shell composed of albumin or galactose. Although these microbubbles were small enough to cross the capillary bed in the lungs, they could not survive the variations in pressure gradients throughout the body. Further improvements were needed in microbubble design in order to increase stability, and second-generation microbubbles were developed. The second-generation microbubbles were filled with a high molecular weight gas to decrease their solubility in the blood, thus increasing their stability and aiding in their survival under pressure gradients.[1] The microbubble shells were further stabilized through the addition of surfactants, albumin, phospholipids, or biodegradable synthetic materials to the shell.[1,2] These improvements in contrast media microbubbles have greatly enhanced the stability and efficacy of these agents for use as ultrasound imaging echo enhancers. Two ultrasound contrast agents are available for use in the United States: Definity (perflutren lipid microsphere injectable suspension [Lantheus]) and Optison (perflutren protein-type A microspheres injectable suspension, USP [GE Healthcare]).

Characteristics of Ultrasound Contrast Microbubbles

For these contrast agents to be effective in enhancing ultrasound imaging, several physical properties are essential for the microbubbles. Table 12-1 lists the key characteristics of an ideal ultrasound contrast agent.

Through the years, changes in the design of ultrasound contrast microbubbles were needed to improve the stability of the microbubbles in circulation and allow them to pass through the pulmonary capillary bed for recirculation. For the microbubbles to be clinically useful and allow systemic enhancement of imaging, they must pass undamaged through the pulmonary, cardiac, and capillary circulations after injection. Microbubbles must be less than 7 µm in diameter to pass through the narrowest capillaries in the body, the pulmonary capillaries.[3,4] Microbubbles most readily oscillate when encountered by an ultrasound signal at a specific frequency that is dependent on their diameter. Fortu-

Table 12-1. Characteristics of an Ideal Ultrasound Contrast Agent

- Must demonstrate the ability to provide bright contrast
- Must be safe and harmless to the patient
- Must be injectable intravenously
- Bubbles should be completely biodegradable and biotolerable
- Presence of bubbles should not affect tissue perfusion
- Bubbles should be broken down by the body and either safely excreted or broken down into products of normal metabolic pathways
- There should be no long-term deposition of the agent or its components in the body
- Bubbles should be stable and robust in vivo
- Bubbles should be retained in the circulation as long as needed to complete the imaging procedure

nately, the resonance frequency of microbubbles with a diameter of less than 7 μm is within the ultrasound frequency range, 2–15 MHz, used for diagnostic imaging.[2,3]

How effective contrast media microbubbles prove to be as echo enhancers for diagnostic ultrasound imaging depends on several factors, such as the microbubble's design, the ultrasound beam acoustic output (power) applied, the frequency transmitted, the reduction of the ultrasound beam with depth, and the signal processing.[5] Microbubbles are much more compressible than tissue. Therefore, when they are exposed to an ultrasound beam they expand and contract, which creates backscatter. The backscatter produced by the microbubbles requires microbubble-specific imaging sequence methods (e.g., harmonic, pulse inversion) for enhancement of the ultrasound images. Because of the specific interactions between the ultrasound beam and the microbubbles, the backscatter signal is greatly increased. This enhancement is most useful in Doppler studies using ultrasound to evaluate blood perfusion. In conventional gray-scale ultrasound imaging, it is not essential to increase the backscatter signal, so contrast is not generally used.[3–5]

At low ultrasound beam power, microbubbles oscillate in a linear fashion. The frequency of the scattered signals is equal to the transmitted frequency. This type of ultrasound imaging is useful for Doppler and real-time perfusion studies. At higher ultrasound beam power, microbubbles oscillate in a nonlinear fashion because they resist compression more than expansion. The scattered signals contain multiples of the transmitted frequency. The higher-frequency parts of the scattered signals are referred to as harmonic signals, which are microbubble specific.[3–5] These microbubble-specific harmonic signals allow favored imaging of the contrast media microbubbles as compared with surrounding tissue, through a nonlinear imaging method such as pulse inversion.[4] At even higher ultrasound beam power, microbubbles break open and diffuse.[3,5] Therefore, depending on the ultrasound beam power used for the imaging procedure, the backscatter signals are processed by microbubble-specific or conventional ultrasound modalities.

The microbubble's shell and gas core enable the contrast agent to be stable in circulation. The shell material affects how the microbubble is handled by the immune system. Depending on the shell composition, immune system cells may take up the microbubbles, identifying them as foreign particles. The external shell is typically composed of denatured albumin, galactose, phospholipids, or polybutyl cyanoacrylate, which may include or exclude surfactants.[4] The shell material also affects the elasticity of the microbubbles. A denatured albumin shell allows the microbubble to be more rigid, whereas a phospholipid shell allows the microbubble to be flexible.[6] The more elastic the shell material, the more energy it can withstand before bursting; this is an important determinant of residence time within the body after intravenous injection, affecting the ability to obtain quality images during an ultrasound study.

The gas core of the current, second-generation ultrasound contrast agents is composed of perfluorocarbon or sulfur hexafluoride. These gases have a high molecular weight, low solubility, and low diffusion coefficient, which allow a high gas concentration inside the microbubble compared with the surrounding blood. This gives the microbubbles increased stability while in circulation.[6] These qualities overcome some of the major issues encountered with earlier-generation contrast agents that used air as the gas core. Air is highly soluble, and leakage from the shell would occur, decreasing the persistence and the stability of the compounds after intravenous injection.

Clinical Applications of Ultrasound Contrast Microbubbles

Ultrasound contrast media microbubbles have many different clinical applications, and many more applications are being developed and tested. Contrast media microbubbles were originally used because they improved Doppler rescue studies—vascular blood flow studies in which tissue attenuation complicates conventional imaging—by increasing the intensity of the signal.[3,4,7] Today, ultrasound studies with contrast-enhanced Doppler are used most commonly in the evaluation of renal and hepatic macrovascular diseases such as stenosis of arteries or veins and microvascular diseases such as infarction and hypoperfusion, and in the detection and description of solid and atypical cystic lesions.[5] Other Doppler rescue studies that use ultrasound contrast agents are evaluation of portal venous patency in cirrhosis, transjugular intrahepatic portosystemic (TIPS) shunts, carotid artery stenosis, liver transplantation, and transcranial Doppler.[7]

Contrast media microbubbles play a significant role in echocardiography. Contrast media in ultrasound imaging is indicated for left-ventricular opacification and to improve definition of the left-ventricular endocardial borders. When contrast media are given to a patient, more precise measurements of left-ventricular volume and ejection fraction have been possible. Contrast media have also been shown to enhance the characterization of structural cardiovascular abnormalities, aid in the diagnosis and grading of cardiac valve disease, and identify complications associated with myocardial infarction.[7]

Oncology is another area in which contrast media have strong clinical applications. Contrast media and specific ultrasound techniques have important applications in liver lesion imaging. Contrast media microbubbles can be used to identify specific enhancement patterns of many different focal liver lesions. Because contrast enhancement patterns are different for benign versus malignant liver lesions, the use of contrast media can help characterize the lesions.[4] Contrast media may also help improve intraoperative ultrasound imaging for the resection of liver metastases. If the patient is not a candidate for resection of the tumor, ablation treatment may be an option, and ultrasound images enhanced by contrast media microbubbles allow the treatment to be completed in fewer sessions, possibly in only a single session.[3,4] Contrast media microbubbles also help to characterize splenic and renal masses.[3,4]

Contrast Agents

Two ultrasound contrast agents are commercially available in the United States: Definity from Lantheus Medical Imaging and Optison from GE Healthcare. The current agents are considered "untargeted" contrast media microbubbles, since they do not diffuse out of circulation; they stay in the intravascular compartment, acting as blood-pool markers.[2,3] This enables information to be obtained regarding vascularity and enhancement features of body tissues.[4] Contrast media microbubbles enable imaging of the anatomy of the macrovasculature and the physiology of the microvasculature.[8] Exciting applications for contrast media microbubbles in gene therapy and targeted drug delivery are currently in the investigational stage. These applications use the contrast microbubbles to carry antibodies, DNA, or drugs to specific tissues or cells in the body, but no such agents are yet available for clinical use.[4]

Definity

Definity (perflutren lipid microsphere injectable suspension) consists of a lipid outer shell, made up of three different phospholipid molecules, surrounding an octofluoropropane (perflutren) gas. The structures of perflutren gas and the phospholipids in the outer shell are shown in Figure 12-1. Definity is used for patients with poor echocardiograms to opacify the left-ventricular chamber and to improve the definition of the left-ventricular endocardial border.[9]

Dosage and Administration

Definity is stored in the refrigerator and must be brought to room temperature before preparation for use. A proprietary device called the Vialmix must be used to activate Definity before administration. This involves agitation for 45 seconds to create a milky-white suspension. The product is ready for use immediately after agitation and can be used for up to 12 hours after initial mixing, with resuspension by using hand agitation for 10 seconds. The product should be activated only once using the Vialmix. Definity may be administered as an intravenous bolus or by intravenous infusion. The recommended bolus dosage is 10 µL/kg within 30–60 seconds, followed by 10 mL of saline flush. A second 10-µL/kg bolus injection followed by a 10-mL saline flush may be given 30 minutes after the first injection if continued contrast enhancement is needed. The recommended infusion dosage is 1.3 mL added to 50 mL of preservative-free saline. The rate of the intravenous infusion is 4 mL/min. The infusion may be adjusted to a maximum rate of 10 mL/min for the best enhancement.[9]

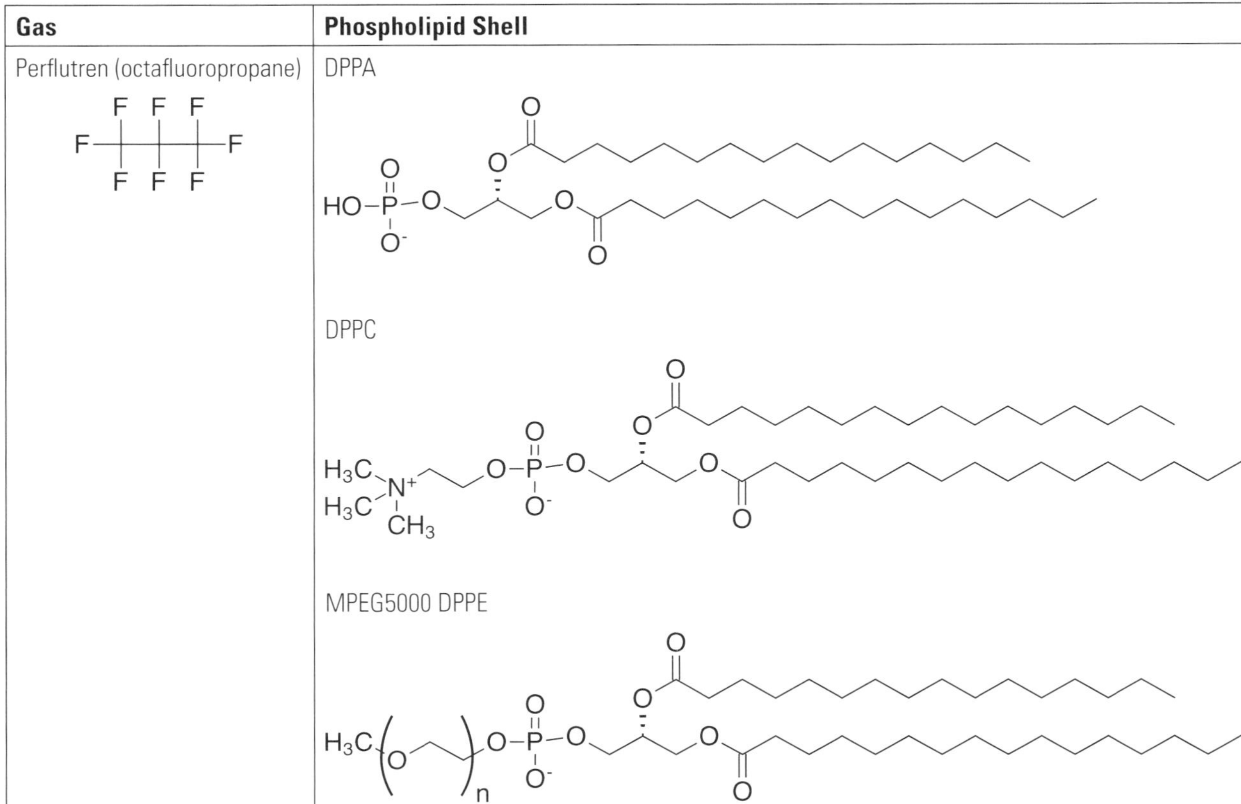

Figure 12-1. Components of Definity (perflutren lipid microsphere injectable suspension from Lantheus).

The pharmacokinetics of the lipid microspheres has not been studied in humans. However, pharmacokinetic information is available for perflutren gas. The gas is stable and is not metabolized by the body. After 10 minutes, perflutren gas was not measurable in the blood or expired air of study patients.[9] The average half-life of perflutren gas was 1.3 minutes in study patients. The phospholipid components of the shell are thought to be metabolized to free fatty acids.[9]

Adverse Reactions

Definity carries the risk of serious cardiopulmonary reactions. Deaths have occurred during or after its administration. Some of the deaths occurred several days after administration and were thought to be attributable to the underlying disease or condition, but the role of Definity as a contributing factor could not be ruled out. Definity carries a black-box warning and should be used with caution in patients with pulmonary hypertension, acute myocardial infarction, acute coronary artery syndromes, worsening or unstable congestive heart failure, serious ventricular arrhythmias, or respiratory failure and in patients receiving mechanical ventilation.[9]

Adverse reactions include injection site reactions, chest pain, and dizziness; the most common adverse reactions are back and renal pain, headache, nausea, and flushing. A small percentage of patients have had adverse reactions requiring discontinuation of drug administration. Most adverse reactions have occurred within the first 15 minutes of administration and have resolved without treatment within minutes to hours after administration. As with all contrast agents, there is potential for hypersensitivity reactions presenting as shock, bronchospasm, laryngeal swelling, urticaria, and pruritus, so patients receiving Definity should be closely monitored during its administration. Drug–drug interactions with Definity have not been studied.[9]

Contraindications

It is contraindicated to administer Definity to patients with possible or known right-to-left, bidirectional, or transient right-to-left cardiac shunts; the reason for this contraindication is to avoid the development of systemic embolization via arterial circulation. Patients with hypersensitivity to perflutren should not receive this agent.[9]

Medication Therapy Management (MTM) Concerns

Definity has a black-box warning for serious cardiopulmonary reactions. The warning states that serious cardiopulmonary reactions, including deaths, have happened during or after the administration of perflutren-containing microspheres. It urges evaluation of all patients for the conditions for which Definity is contraindicated. The warning suggests monitoring vital signs, electrocardiography, and cutaneous oxygen saturation in patients with pulmonary hypertension or unstable cardiopulmonary conditions. This should be done during and for at least 30 minutes after administration of Definity. Trained medical personnel and proper resuscitation equipment need to be accessible in case of an emergency.[9]

Although there is a black-box warning on this product, many professionals in the field of diagnostic imaging think this warning does not accurately reflect the efficacy and established safety profile of the ultrasound contrast agents, the potential risk of other procedures, and the effect of the *pseudocomplication*—defined as a complication after any medical procedure that may be caused by the procedure or by development of the underlying disease. These professionals believe pseudocomplications are the reason for many adverse events associated with ultrasound contrast agents, and they suggest that the black-box warning about ultrasound contrast agents containing perflutren be removed.[10]

Optison

The Optison microbubble suspension consists of a microsphere component called protein-type A, with a human serum albumin component,[11] combined with the gas perflutren (see structure in Figure 12-1). Optison is indicated for patients with poor echocardiograms to opacify the left-ventricular chamber and to improve the definition of the left-ventricular endocardial border.[11]

Dosage and Administration

Optison is stored in the refrigerator and must be gently inverted and rotated to resuspend the microspheres. This is done until the vial comes to room temperature and the particles are completely resuspended. The solution will be an opaque milky-white color when completely resuspended. Optison is drawn into an injection syringe and is administered as an intravenous bolus injection into a peripheral vein. The recommended dose is 0.5 mL to be injected no faster than 1 mL/sec, but with the injection time not exceeding 1 minute. If the injection is not complete within 1 minute, the remaining material in the syringe needs to be resuspended by gentle rotation and inversion. The bolus dose is followed by a 10-mL saline or 5% dextrose flush. If more contrast enhancement is needed after the initial dose, additional 0.5-mL incremental doses may be administered, up to 5 mL in a 10-minute period. There is a maximum total dose of 8.7 mL in any one patient study.[11]

The pharmacokinetics of neither the microspheres nor the human albumin component has been studied in humans. However, pharmacokinetic information is available for perflutren gas. The gas is stable and is not metabolized by the body. After 10 minutes, most of the perflutren gas was expired through the lungs in study patients.[11] The average half-life of perflutren gas was 1.3 minutes in the study patients. The human albumin component of the shell is thought to be metabolized by the typical method for human albumin.[11]

Adverse Reactions

Because the administration of Optison can lead to serious cardiopulmonary reactions, possibly including death, this agent carries a black-box warning. Optison should be used with caution in patients with pulmonary hypertension, acute myocardial infarction, acute coronary artery syndromes, worsening or unstable congestive heart failure, serious ventricular arrhythmias, or respiratory failure and in patients receiving mechanical ventilation.[11]

More common adverse reactions include headache, warm sensation/flushing, chills/fever, flulike symptoms, malaise/weakness/fatigue, dizziness, chest pain, nausea/vomiting, dyspnea, injection site discomfort, erythema, and altered taste. There is potential for acute anaphylactoid reactions following administration of this agent, even in patients who have had no prior exposure to perflutren-containing microspheres. All patients should be monitored for signs and symptoms of these types of reactions. Drug–drug interactions with Optison have not been studied.[11]

Contraindications

It is contraindicated to administer Optison to patients with possible or known right-to-left, bidirectional, or transient right-to-left cardiac shunts; the reason for this contraindication is to avoid the development of systemic embolization via arterial circulation. Patients with hypersensitivity to perflutren, blood, blood products, or albumin also should not receive this agent.[11]

MTM Concerns

Optison has a black-box warning for serious cardiopulmonary reactions. The warning states that serious cardiopulmonary reactions, including deaths, have happened during or after the administration of perflutren-containing microspheres. It urges evaluation of all patients for the conditions for which Optison is contraindicated. The warning suggests monitoring vital signs, electrocardiography, and cutaneous oxygen saturation in patients with pulmonary hypertension or unstable cardiopulmonary conditions. This should be done during and for at least 30 minutes after administration of Optison. Trained medical personnel and proper resuscitation equipment need to be accessible in case of an emergency.[11]

Although there is a black-box warning on this product, many professionals in the field of diagnostic imaging think this warning does not accurately reflect the efficacy and established safety profile of the ultrasound contrast agents, the potential risk of other procedures, and the effect of the pseudocomplication (defined above). These professionals believe pseudocomplications are the reason for many adverse events associated with ultrasound contrast agents, and they suggest that the black-box warning about ultrasound contrast agents containing perflutren be removed.[10]

Since Optison contains albumin, there is a possibility for transmission of viral disease, although the risk is remote. There have been no reports of any cases of transmission by this or any other albumin-containing product.

Conclusion

Contrast media microbubbles for ultrasound imaging act as echo enhancers that increase the backscatter signal by >300-fold,[4] thus improving Doppler analysis and gray-scale echo structure.[5] Contrast media ultrasound may be more convenient and cost-effective than computed tomography (CT) and magnetic resonance imaging (MRI), and comparable to CT and MRI in certain diagnostic imaging situations. Contrast media microbubbles can be delivered and processed under real-time ultrasound observation.[3,4] Contrast media microbubbles are well tolerated by patients; severe adverse effects are infrequent.[4] Although the contrast media agents for ultrasound imaging carry a black-box warning, many professionals in the field do not believe the warning to be appropriate. Contrast media microbubbles for ultrasound imaging have many important clinical applications today and many potential applications in the future. They appear to be effective, safe, and well tolerated by patients.

References

1. Dijkmans PA, Juffermans LJM, Musters RJP, et al. Microbubbles and ultrasound: from diagnosis to therapy. *Eur J Echocardiography.* 2004;5:245–56.
2. Calliada F, Campani R, Bottinelli O, et al. Ultrasound contrast agents: basic principles. *Eur J Radiol.* 1998;27(suppl):S157–S160.
3. Cosgrove D. Ultrasound contrast agents: an overview. *Eur J Radiol.* 2006;60: 324–30.
4. Stewart VR, Sidhu PS. New directions in ultrasound: microbubble contrast. *Br J Radiol.* 2006;79:188–94. http://bjr.birjournals.org/cgi/content/full/79/939/188. Accessed August 17, 2011.
5. Correas JM, Bridal L, Lesavre A, et al. Ultrasound contrast agents: properties, principles of action, tolerance, and artifacts. *Eur Radiol.* 2001;11:1316–28.
6. Quaia E. Microbubble ultrasound contrast agents: an update. *Eur Radiol.* 2007;17: 1995–2008.
7. Harvey CJ, Blomley MJK, Eckersley RJ, et al. Developments in ultrasound contrast media. *Eur Radiol.* 2001;11:675–89.
8. Feinstein SB. The powerful microbubble: from bench to bedside, from intravascular indicator to therapeutic delivery system, and beyond. *Am J Physiol Heart Circ Physiol.* 2004;287:H450–H457.
9. Definity [package insert]. North Billerica, MA: Lantheus Medical Imaging; 2008.
10. Main ML, Grayburn PA, Goldman JH, et al. Presentation to the Food and Drug Administration Cardiovascular and Renal Drugs Advisory Committee regarding safety considerations in the development of ultrasound contrast agents. www.fda.gov/ohrms/dockets/ac/08/slides/2008-4369s1-12-OPH_files/slide0995.htm. Accessed March 18, 2010.
11. Optison [package insert]. Princeton, NJ: GE Healthcare; 2008.

CHAPTER 13

Regulations Associated with the Use of Ionizing Radiation

Mack L. Richard and Kara D. Weatherman

The use of ionizing radiation for medical diagnostic procedures has recently received a significant amount of public attention. The question being raised is whether the potential long-term risks of repeated exposure to ionizing radiation through diagnostic testing are greater than the long-term benefits derived.[1–3] Those on each side of this discussion have strong opinions. Furthermore, the words "radioactivity" and "nuclear" often have negative connotations, giving many people a level of unease about undergoing a diagnostic test that involves ionizing radiation. Although most pharmacists have a limited background in the area of radiation safety, they are often in a position to counsel patients about their medical care. This chapter presents an overview of the potential for radiation exposure of patients and personnel and the policies and regulations that are in place to ensure patient and employee safety throughout the diagnostic imaging process. The controversy over the risks versus the benefits of ionizing radiation is discussed briefly to help pharmacists formulate their own opinions on the subject and counsel patients and family members on these topics.

Regulatory Oversight

The use of radioactive materials for diagnostic imaging is highly regulated in regard to not only the risk to patients undergoing imaging procedures but also the risk to medical professionals who are exposed during the imaging process. Which regulatory agencies govern the use of ionizing radiation in medical imaging is determined by the source of the radiation. Imaging devices that use machine-produced radiation primarily include radiographic (x-ray) units, fluoroscopic units, and computed tomography (CT) scanners. These types of imaging devices and the personnel who operate them are regulated by the individual states. With other types of imaging (nuclear medicine and positron-emission tomography [PET]), images are generated from radiation as it is emitted from the body of a patient who has been administered radioactive material. The use of radioactive materials for these imaging applications is regulated either by the federal Nuclear Regulatory Commission (NRC) or by a regulatory agency in a state that has entered into an agreement with NRC (i.e., an "agreement state") to develop, implement, and enforce regulations consistent with NRC regulations. Currently, 37 of the 50 states are agreement states.[4] Thus, for medical facilities that use radioactive materials in agreement states, the regulatory authority rests with a state agency, whereas for the remaining states such medical facilities are regulated by NRC. The individual agreement state or NRC is responsible for issuing radioactive material licenses to medical facilities for the use of such materials. These licenses designate the various radioactive materials that can be possessed, how those materials can be used, and any specific conditions associated with their use.

NRC or the agreement state has broad oversight regarding the safe possession and use of radioactive materials in medical applications. Agreement states are responsible for developing their own set of standards, but these are closely related to the NRC requirements for the safe handling and use of ionizing radiation in both diagnostic and therapeutic applications. The NRC standards are found in the Code of Federal Regulations (CFR), primarily in Title 10 CFR Part 35, concerning medical use of radiation.[5] These extensive regulations cover all aspects of the handling and use of radioactive materials for medical purposes.

NRC and state agencies are also responsible for regulating the manufacture and distribution of radiation-emitting products, in partnership with the Food and Drug Administration, and they work closely with state regulatory agencies overseeing the practices of both medicine and pharmacy to ensure the safety and quality of the radioactive materials used in humans. NRC's Advisory Committee on the Medical Uses of Isotopes (ACMUI) consists of members of the health care professions who provide feedback to NRC on current trends and issues dealing with the medical use of radiation.[6]

Regulatory Compliance and the Radiation Safety Officer (RSO)

Facilities that use radiation or radioactive materials are typically required by regulation or licensure conditions to identify an individual who is responsible for ensuring compliance with the appropriate state or NRC regulations and licensure conditions. That individual is usually called the radiation safety officer (RSO) or radiation protection officer. In large medical institutions that use many different types of radioactive materials or use those materials for both diagnostic and therapeutic procedures, the RSO typically is an individual who has received specific training in health physics (radiation protection) and devotes his or her entire effort to ensuring compliance with regulations and licensure conditions. In these large institutions, the RSO often has additional professionally or technically trained staff to assist in the implementation of the radiation safety program. Conversely, in smaller medical facilities, the individual named as the RSO may be someone whose primary responsibility is not radiation protection but who has sufficient training and experience with radioactive materials to serve as the RSO. In these smaller medical facilities, a nuclear medicine physician, a medical physicist, or perhaps a nuclear pharmacist may serve as the RSO.

The RSO is required to implement appropriate policies and procedures and perform evaluations to ensure that all regulations and licensure conditions are being met. Furthermore, most regulatory agencies require that the management of the facility provide a written "delegation of authority" to the RSO, granting him or her the authority to take appropriate actions (including the suspension of radioactive material use) to ensure compliance with the regulations and licensure conditions. In larger institutions, a radiation safety committee is required by regulation to be established to provide adequate support for the RSO.

Major Sources of Radiation Exposure

As background for a discussion of the potential effects of radiation exposure, it is necessary to understand the standards used to quantify the amount of radiation (dose) that a patient receives. The SI unit Sievert (Sv) or the metric unit roentgen equivalent in man (rem) is used to express radiation doses. To convert between the units, 1 Sv = 100 rem.[7] In the United States, radiation doses are most often reported in rem, whereas Sv is used widely throughout the remainder of the world.

Radiation is present all around us, and every person has some degree of exposure to radiation. The average annual radiation dose in the United States is 620 mrem (6.2 mSv), coming from both natural and artificially produced sources.[8] Naturally occurring radiation can be cosmic or terrestrial. A person's exposure to background radiation varies greatly by geographic location and the types of material with which the person has regular contact. People living at higher altitudes have a greater amount of cosmic radiation exposure than people living at lower altitudes. Materials such as brick, stone, and granite have higher radiation levels than wood. About half of the total radiation exposure a person receives in a year comes from naturally occurring sources.[8,9] The average annual radiation exposure from naturally occurring radiation sources is 310 mrem, or 3.1 mSv; two-thirds of this comes from radioactive gases such as radon, with the remainder coming from cosmic, terrestrial, and other types of radiation.

Exposure to man-made (artificial) types of radiation from medical diagnostic imaging and from commercial and industrial sources makes up the other half of the average person's annual radiation dose, accounting for 310 mrem (3.1 mSv). Averaged over one's lifetime, medical imaging procedures account for about 300 mrem (3.0 mSv), or 97% of the total exposure from man-made sources. Of those medical exposures, CT scans account for about 147 mrem (1.47 mSv), nuclear medicine imaging procedures for approximately 77 mrem (0.77 mSv), and interventional fluoroscopy and conventional radiography/fluoroscopy for about 76 mrem (0.76 mSv)—or about 47%, 25%, and 25%, respectively, of the total average exposure from man-made sources. The remainder is from consumer products such as tobacco, fertilizer, luminous watch dials, and smoke detectors.[9]

NRC limits the radiation dose allowable over and above the 620 mrem annual average. The NRC annual limit for occupational radiation exposure is 5000 mrem (50 mSv) for personnel such as nuclear pharmacists and nuclear medicine technologists and 100 mrem (1 mSv) for individual members of the public.[10]

Risk of Exposure from Diagnostic Procedures

The amount of ionizing radiation exposure through diagnostic imaging procedures depends on the type of procedure and the duration of the patient's exposure to the radioactive source. Using the lowest possible amount of radiation necessary to perform a given imaging procedure is thought to keep patient risk to a minimum. Studies have shown a statistically significant increase in the risk for leukemia and other cancers in individuals who have received effective radiation doses in excess of 10 rem (100 mSv) delivered in a relatively short period of time.[11] No studies published to date have proven a direct causal relationship between medical imaging and an increased risk of cancer; most risk estimates are based on data from significant radiation exposures such as in the atomic bombing of Japan, accidents at nuclear reactors, and the early use of x-rays. Although the effective dose from medical imaging procedures varies considerably, rarely does a patient receive more than 2000 mrem (20 mSv). Table 13-1 lists average adult radiation doses from common diagnostic imaging procedures.[12] (For comparison, the table also shows the average radiation dose from a whole-body airport security scan—another controversial use of radiation.[13]) Of course, a patient may undergo multiple medical imaging procedures over time and, even if the effective dose from a single procedure is well below 10 rem (100 mSv), the cumulative effective dose for multiple procedures could approach or exceed that amount.

Some individuals and organizations believe that any radiation exposure poses a risk. Despite the lack of definitive studies showing an increased risk of cancer in individuals receiving an effective dose of less than 10 rem (100 mSv), they take the position that it is prudent to assume that some risk exists. This is referred to the "linear no-threshold hypothesis." Some studies have suggested that exposure to radiation during medical imaging may be responsible for 1% to 3% of all cancers worldwide.[13] Thus, it is important that medical imaging procedures be performed only if the information obtained from the procedure provides a specific benefit to the patient that outweighs any increased risk from the radiation effective dose associated

Table 13-1. Average Adult Radiation Dose from Common Diagnostic Imaging Procedures[11,12]

Study	Radiation Dose (mSv)
Plain film chest x-ray	0.10
Plain film abdominal x-ray	0.70
Plain film extremity x-ray (arm, leg)	0.01
Plain film mammogram	0.40
Plain film panoramic dental x-ray	0.01
Chest CT (standard)	7.0
Chest CT (pulmonary embolism)	15.0
Cardiac CT	16.0
Abdomen CT (standard)	8.0
Abdomen/pelvis CT	14.0
Virtual colonoscopy	10.0
Upper GI fluoroscopy	6.0
Barium enema fluoroscopy	8.0
Nuclear medicine lung scan	2.2
Nuclear medicine cardiac stress test (^{99m}Tc)	9.4
Nuclear medicine gallbladder scan	3.1
Nuclear medicine renal scan	2.6
Nuclear medicine bone scan	6.3
Nuclear medicine white blood cell study	6.7
Nuclear medicine thyroid scan	4.8
PET whole-body scan	14.1
Coronary angiogram (diagnostic)	7.0
Coronary angiogram (stent placement)	15.0
Airport security whole-body scan	0.0001[13]

with the procedure. Another concern relates to the exposure of children to radiation for imaging. Since studies have shown that the risk from radiation exposure is higher for children than for adults, special emphasis must be placed on minimizing radiation doses to children from imaging procedures.

With certain imaging procedures, the duration of radiation exposure can increase the patient's risk for adverse effects other than cancer. For example, fluoroscopy may be used to generate continuous x-rays during a procedure such as the insertion of a catheter into a coronary vessel. Particularly if complications arise during the procedure, long fluoroscopy times can result in radiation doses to the skin high enough to cause erythema (skin reddening) where the x-ray beam enters the patient. Although rare, a few cases have been documented in which very high fluoroscopy doses have resulted in more severe skin effects, including ulceration and skin necrosis that required skin grafts.[14]

In some instances it may be necessary to calculate the radiation dose to a patient. One such instance is when a female patient learns after an imaging procedure that she was pregnant at the time of the procedure. Another is when the wrong radiopharmaceutical has been administered to a patient. In such cases, a health physicist or medical physicist may be called upon to calculate the radiation dose to the conceptus of the pregnant female or to the patient who received the incorrect radiopharmaceutical. Depending upon the regulatory requirements, it may be necessary to notify a regulatory agency if the calculated dose exceeds a certain level.

Optimization

The individual primarily responsible for patient safety in medical imaging is the physician (the nuclear medicine physician or the radiologist). However, all individuals involved in the performance of an imaging procedure (nuclear medicine technologists, radiographers, and if applicable, radiopharmacists) share this responsibility. Their goal is to provide the best images with the smallest amount of radiation exposure for the patient. This is sometimes referred to as "optimization." To achieve optimization, imaging protocols and procedures should be developed to ensure that the patient receives the lowest possible radiation dose for obtaining the necessary images. Imaging protocols should be tailored to the patient. Quality assurance procedures should be followed to ensure that imaging devices are operating properly. Training programs for individuals performing the imaging procedures are particularly important as new imaging technology becomes available. Periodic refresher training is also recommended and sometimes required by regulation for individuals performing and supervising the procedures.

Preventing and Monitoring Occupational Exposure

All users of radiation also have a responsibility to protect themselves, their co-workers, and members of the general public from unnecessary radiation exposures. The primary factors in reducing external exposure to radiation are time, distance, and shielding. Individuals should minimize the time they spend in close proximity to sources of radiation, including patients who have received radiopharmaceuticals. They should maximize the distance between themselves and the radiation source. External radiation exposure follows the inverse square law; doubling the distance from a radiation source decreases exposure by a factor of four. Shielding is used to absorb the radiation energy and prevent exposure of the user. Shielding commonly used in radiology departments includes lead aprons to protect the trunk of the body, lead collars to protect the thyroid gland, and lead glasses to protect the eyes from scattered x-rays during fluoroscopy procedures in which medical staff may have to be in close proximity to the patient. Imaging rooms where x-rays are generated are evaluated by a health physicist or medical physicist to ensure that proper shielding is included in the walls to protect individuals in surrounding areas. In nuclear medicine departments, lead syringe and vial shields are used to reduce radiation exposure of personnel to radiopharmaceuticals before administration to patients. Bench-top shields are used by nuclear medicine technologists drawing up individual doses from multidose vials. Similar types of shields are found in PET imaging areas; however, because of the higher-energy annihilation radiation emitted by PET radiopharmaceuticals, thicker lead shields are required.

The preparation and administration of radiopharmaceuticals involves the handling of unsealed sources (usually liquids) that may contaminate the individuals handling these materials or contaminate the work area. It is important that appropriate barrier controls such as disposable gloves and lab coats or other long-sleeved garments be used to minimize personal contamination. Individuals who handle unsealed sources of radioactive material should periodically survey their hands and clothing with an appropriate survey device (e.g., Geiger counter) to detect any contamination and quickly remove it. Appropriate surveys should also be performed to detect contamination of laboratory surfaces, and proper decontamination procedures should be used when necessary. Using such contamination control methods minimizes the likelihood of skin contamination or internal contamination from ingestion or inhalation.

It is important that a monitoring program be established to measure the external radiation exposure of occupationally exposed individuals, as well as any internal contamination that may occur. Depending upon the potential for external exposure, devices may be issued to individuals for monitoring whole-body or hand exposure from various radiation sources. If internal contamination is anticipated or suspected, a bioassay program may be implemented to measure the internal deposition of radioactive material and calculate the resulting effective dose. Usually, the RSO or radiation safety committee evaluates the need for personnel monitoring or bioassays.

Radiation protection in the medical environment follows the principle of keeping radiation doses to both patients and medical staff as low as reasonably achievable, or ALARA. The overall radiation safety program in a medical facility should be designed to ensure that the ALARA principle is being implemented.

Minimizing the Effective Dose to Patients

Since some degree of risk may exist for any patient exposed to radiation in the course of a diagnostic imaging procedure, it is essential that practitioners ordering such procedures weigh that risk against the benefit of information to be obtained from the procedure. Unfortunately, not all physicians are knowledgeable about the relative risks of various imaging procedures, and the desire to use a more advanced imaging technology may take precedence over the use of a procedure that provides a lower radiation dose.

The number of CT scans performed on adults in the United States increased from approximately 3 million in 1980 to more than 62 million in 2007, and at least 4 million scans were performed on children.[15] Much of this increase was due to the increasing number of CT scanners available and advances in CT technology that have made the acquisition of information extremely easy for the patient, the technologist, and the ordering physician. The greatest increase in the use of CT has been as a screening technology (in the absence of definitive patient symptoms) rather than as a diagnostic technology (in symptomatic patients).[16,17] Screening applications in adults have included CT colonoscopy (also called virtual colonoscopy), CT lung screening for smokers, CT cardiac screening, and whole-body CT screening. Although CT use in pediatric populations has also increased significantly, most often it is for diagnostic purposes.[18,19] Another factor in the increased use of CT scanning has been defensive medicine, in which physicians tend to order studies to cover all bases when a diagnosis does not readily present itself. Lack of communication between health care providers can also contribute to the overuse of scanning; a patient may have multiple tests ordered by different physicians who do not have access to the patient's full medical record and do not know what tests have previously been performed.

Although CT scanning is an essential tool in many instances, there is increasing evidence that many physicians order CT scanning unnecessarily because they view it as having the same risk level as any other type of imaging, not considering that a procedure using less radiation or no radiation at all could be used instead. A survey of patients, radiologists, and emergency room physicians to determine their awareness of the radiation dose and relative risk associated with CT scanning revealed a general lack of knowledge and understanding by all parties.[20] Only 7% of the patients (5 of 76 surveyed) had been informed about potential risks and benefits of their CT scan. Regarding the potential increased cancer risk, 47% of the radiologists (18 of 38 surveyed) acknowledged the possibility, whereas only 9% of the emergency room physicians (4 of 45 surveyed) and 3% of patients (3 of 76 surveyed) believed there was an increased risk. Most of the physicians and none of the patients were able to accurately estimate the difference between the radiation dose from a single CT study and that from a single chest x-ray.

Given these findings, what steps can be taken to reduce the radiation dose from diagnostic imaging studies? Physicians should carefully consider the need to order not only CT studies but any procedure that uses ionizing radiation. If physicians stop ordering studies when they are not necessary, this could drastically reduce the total radiation dose to patients. A diagnostic imaging procedure may be justified by the patient's medical condition and working diagnosis, as the potential benefit may outweigh the risk. However, some reviews have indicated that as many as one-third of the CT studies that are ordered could be either eliminated or replaced by an imaging procedure that does not use ionizing radiation.[21] If that is true, judicious evaluation of the need to perform a study with ionizing radiation would prevent as many as 20 million adults and 1 million pediatric patients, based on current utilization patterns, from receiving an unnecessary radiation dose.

As technology advances, so do the quality and safety features of the imaging equipment. Many of the newer CT scanners have automatic exposure control options to limit the total dose administered to a patient during a study. However, such features are not foolproof. At two facilities in California excessive doses of radiation, including a significant overdose in a pediatric patient, resulted from inappropriate use of imaging equipment.[1]

Another option for decreasing exposure is to switch from a procedure that uses ionizing radiation to one that does not. Ultrasound and magnetic resonance imaging do not use ionizing radiation. As technology improves in these areas, the diagnostic information obtained may be as good as or better than that obtained with a CT scan.

Conclusion

The level of regulatory oversight of facilities and personnel handling, interacting with, and administering doses of ionizing radiation is considerable. Its purpose is to ensure the safety of both patients and the workers who are regularly exposed to radiation. Although the risk of radiation-induced damage as a result of diagnostic imaging is not entirely clear, each decision to use these imaging technologies should include an evaluation of their safety. Continual review of data on the use of ionizing radiation will help ensure the safe and effective use of imaging procedures for patients in the future.

References

1. Bogdanich W. Radiation overdoses point up dangers of CT scans. *New York Times.* October 15, 2009.
2. Chan A. Mammogram benefit outweighs risks, study finds. Live Science. November 16, 2010. www.livescience.com/8970-mammogram-benefits-outweigh-radiation-risks-study-finds.html. Accessed August 2011.
3. Fazel R, Krumholz H, Wang Y, et al. Exposure to low-dose ionizing radiation from medical imaging procedures. *N Engl J Med.* 2009;361:849–57.

4. US Nuclear Regulatory Commission. Agreement state program. www.nrc.gov/about-nrc/state-tribal/agreement-states.html. Accessed June 2011.
5. 10 CFR Part 35.
6. US Nuclear Regulatory Commission. Advisory Committee on the Medical Use of Isotopes. www.nrc.gov/about-nrc/regulatory/advisory/acmui.html. Accessed June 2011.
7. Thompson A, Taylor B. Guide for the use of the international system of units (SI). NIST Special Publication 811. Gaithersburg, MD: National Institute of Standards and Technology, US Department of Commerce; March 2008.
8. US Nuclear Regulatory Commission. Fact sheet on biological effects of radiation. www.nrc.gov/reading-rm/doc-collections/fact-sheets/bio-effects-radiation.html. Accessed June 2011.
9. Ionizing Radiation Exposure of the Population of the United States. Report no. 160. Bethesda, MD: National Council on Radiation Protection and Measurements; 2009.
10. 10 CFR part 20.
11. National Research Council of the National Academies. *Health Risks from Exposure to Low Levels of Ionizing Radiation. BEIR VII Phase 2.* http://books.nap.edu/catalog/11340.html. Accessed June 2011.
12. Mettler FA Jr, Huda W, Yoshizumi TT, et al. Effective doses in radiology and diagnostic nuclear medicine: a catalog. *Radiology.* 2008:248;254–63.
13. American College of Radiology. ACR statement on airport full-body scanners and radiation. January 2010. www.acr.org/mainmenucategories/media_room/featuredcategories/pressreleases/statementonairportfullbodyscanners.aspx. Accessed June 2011.
14. Koenig TR, Mettler FA, Wagner LK. Skin injuries from fluoroscopically guided procedures: part 2, review of 73 cases and recommendations for minimizing dose delivered to patient. *AJR Am J Roentgenol.* 2001;177:13–20.
15. Brenner DJ, Hall EJ. Computed tomography—an increasing source of radiation exposure. *N Engl J Med.* 2007;357:2277–84.
16. Brenner DJ, Georgsson MA. Mass screening with CT colonography: should the radiation exposure be of concern? *Gastroenterology.* 2005;129:328–37.
17. Brenner DJ. Radiation risks potentially associated with low-dose CT screening of adult smokers for lung cancer. *Radiology.* 2004;231:440–5.
18. White KS. Helical/spiral CT scanning: a pediatric radiology perspective. *Pediatr Radiol.* 1996;26:5–14.
19. Linton OW, Mettler FA. National conference on dose reduction in CT, with an emphasis on pediatric patients. *AJR Am J Roentgenol.* 2003;181:321–9.
20. Lee CI, Haims AH, Monico EP, et al. Diagnostic CT scans: assessment of patient, physician, and radiologist awareness of radiation dose and possible risks. *Radiology.* 2004;231:393–8.
21. Slovis TL, Berdon WE. Panel discussion. *Pediatr Radiol.* 2002;32:242–4.

Index

Page numbers followed by *f* or *t* indicate figures or tables, respectively.

A

H

I

N

S

U